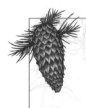

This book is a gift from:

Judith Anne Desjardins

Praise for *Our Journey with Prostate Cancer*

"*From the initial shock of diagnosis and handling the emotions that affect individuals, families, and circles of friends to weighing prostate cancer treatment options and results,* Our Journey with Prostate Cancer *provides plenty of medical and spiritual insights and considers the entire process of recovery to include spiritual development; not just those surrounding treatment options and alternative therapies…*

***Judith Anne Desjardins has created a unique chronicle in the annals of cancer experience and research** by incorporating a range of multi-faceted approaches to handling cancer and its challenges, juxtaposing perspectives from journal entries (by not only herself but others), and creating an atmosphere of positive honesty: one which provides concrete images, approaches, and insights…*

***Any reader interested in choosing empowerment over illness** will find* Our Journey with Prostate Cancer *an inviting, easy and thought-provoking read, filled with a variety of reflections, strategies and options!*"

MIDWEST BOOK REVIEW
(D. DONOVAN, SENIOR e-BOOK REVIEWER)

"Don't let "Prostate" in the title cause you to think you or a loved one suffering from prostate cancer are the only ones I would recommend this book to. **The journey that takes place in this book is well worth the read even if you, your loved one, a family member or a friend don't even have cancer of any kind.**

All the suggestions mentioned in the book and the experiences movingly documented in journal entries apply to all of life's difficulties... The suggestions are practical guides to living life to the fullest by carefully administering to the needs of body, minds, hearts and souls..."

ALLBOOKS REVIEW (PETER KLEIN)

"Our Journey with Prostate Cancer *by Judith Anne Desjardins provides a thorough description of the entire journey of prostate cancer, and can be easily applied to any type of cancer.*

Not only was this book incredibly informative by providing detailed descriptions of many processes, treatments, stages of emotions, and other important information, it is also a comfort to know that others are going through the same struggles. I will keep this book for future reference because cancer is a very real possibility for every family. Thank you for writing this book and sharing your journey of this experience.

I am changed from reading this book and I know everyone who reads this book will find comfort and healing. I recommend this book to anyone wanting to be informed of the journey of cancer."

READER VIEWS (CHRISTINE WATSON)

"For anyone, writing a book about a private, personal battle with an illness would be a momentous task. But to write a book about a personal experience and turn it into an advice guide for others is quite a serious challenge. Judith Anne Desjardins was more than ready for this challenge after she published her true account of her husband's battle with prostate cancer...

Her advice is not simply from her husband's battle with illness but it is knowledge she gained working with patients, doctors, nurses, and patients' family members. She is able to key in on the human psyche and mental capacity so well and it shows beautifully in these guides...

In this heart-felt book, Judith Anne Desjardins opens the door and allows the readers to enter a world full of hope..."

PACIFIC BOOK REVIEW (TIFFANY EZUMA)

Also by Judith Anne Desjardins

Creating A Healthy Life and Marriage; A Holistic Approach: Body, Mind, Emotions and Spirit, Spirit House Publishing, 2010.

Zranione Serca (Polish translation of *Creating A Healthy Life*), published by Purana Publishing, 2013.

our journey

with

prostate cancer

EMPOWERING STRATEGIES for PATIENTS and FAMILIES

JUDITH ANNE DESJARDINS
LCSW, BCD, MSWAC
Award-winning author of *Creating a Healthy Life & Marriage*

Spirit House Publishing

SANTA MONICA, CALIFORNIA
SpiritHousePub.com

OUR JOURNEY WITH PROSTATE CANCER

Spirit House Publishing
3435 Ocean Park Blvd., #107-418
Santa Monica, CA 90405
www.SpiritHousePub.com

Book design by TLC Graphics
Cover by Tamara Dever/Interior Design by Erin Stark

Cover photo credit: ID 22048917 © Sergiyn | Dreamstime.com
Interior graphics credits: Pen image © Depositphotos.com/mishoo

ISBN: 978-0-9904994-0-4

Library of Congress Control Number: 2014910734

First Edition

10 9 8 7 6 5 4 3 2 1

Printed in the United States of America

Disclaimer: The recommendations suggested in this book are not intended as a substitute for consulting with your physician. All matters concerning your health require medical supervision. Neither the author nor the publisher shall be liable or responsible for any loss or damage allegedly arising from any information or recommendations in this book.

Dedication

For My Husband – My Inspiration
*Your warrior spirit courses
throughout the pages of this book.*

For the Men Around the World
Who Are Living With Prostate Cancer
and for Their Loved Ones
We are with you in solidarity and love.

In Memory and Tribute

O. Carl Simonton, M.D.

1942 – 2009

*Thank you for your groundbreaking research into
the mind-body-emotions connection in treating cancer.
Training with you changed the course of my life.*

Irene Watson

1946 – 2012

*You were my literary mentor and my friend.
You are a testimony of love, courage,
defiance, strength and service.*

Louis Zamperini

1917 – 2014

*Your unbreakable spirit gave us courage
on our darkest days. You inspire men
and women around the world.*

Table of Contents

Acknowledgements

+ My husband's prostate cancer was detected through routine digital rectal exams (DREs) and PSA screenings by his urologist. Because these procedures were done on a yearly or twice-a-year basis, changes were noticed from the baseline and a biopsy was recommended. Had these procedures not been done, my husband's high-risk prostate cancer would have silently progressed to Stage IV and possible death.

+ Although my husband is the major contributor to this book, he has chosen to withhold his name.

+ I wish to thank my neighbor, Naples, Italy-born Catarina Fusco. She is a strong prayer warrior who prayed for me and my husband every day for a year. Her love and prayers were invaluable and sustained me during the darkest period of our journey.

+ My colleague Jill Wilson encouraged me to write this book in the early stages of my journaling. She gave me encouragement, clinical suggestions and recommendations, and honest feedback. She was my "link to the outside world" and kept gently prodding me forward. Her love and prayers were constant and a great source of strength, when I needed them the most.

✦ Publishing a book can be an arduous task. My book design team from TLC Graphics was a true gift from God —composed of people who made my manuscript "baby" come to life in the gentlest and most joyful manner. Each person on the team is an expert in their field: Tamara Dever, gifted cover designer and team shepherd; Peter Vogt, my editor who challenged me with questions that required me to dig deep within myself, and who pushed me to develop certain sections and concepts; Erin Stark, master of interior design and creativity whose beautiful interior softened the seriousness of the content. Working with each of them was a healing, loving experience.

✦ Last and certainly not least, my thanks to God, who has sustained me throughout my life and who led and strengthened my husband and me every step of our journey.

Introduction

IN JUNE 1976 I WAS SITTING IN A GROUP INTERVIEW, MAKing my bid for the coveted position of first oncology social worker at St. John's Hospital in Santa Monica, California. I had flown in from Phoenix, Arizona, where I was working as the first psychiatric social worker in the St. Joseph's Hospital inpatient psychiatric unit. I had seen this new job posted in the Sunday edition of the *Los Angeles Times* and had called on Monday to request an interview.

I was told that the social service staff had already narrowed the field to the best candidates, and that they were planning to make their final decision about who to hire on Tuesday. As a courtesy, though, the staff members agreed to see me on Monday. Pleased with my initial presentation, they invited me to return on Tuesday for an intensive group interview. Toward the end of the hour one of the staff members asked me: "What makes you feel you are the best candidate for the job?"

I paused a moment before I responded, knowing that what I was about to say might be controversial. I swallowed hard and gave my answer: "In my two years working on the medicine and neurology units at Maricopa General Hospital in Phoenix, I learned the importance of interdisciplinary teamwork in the delivery of care to the patients. With stroke patients, I learned the need for intensive patient involvement and motivation in recovering movement and speech." So far so good; the staff members were nodding their approval.

"In my year at the St. Joseph's inpatient psychiatric unit," I continued, "I've been the first psychiatric social worker and have had the opportunity to define and develop that role. I've worked extensively with patients who have been immobilized by major depression, and I've developed many techniques for assisting them. I've done intensive individual therapy, family therapy, and group therapy. I've worked with a team of psychiatrists and psychiatric nurses and coordinated the weekly patient assessment meetings.

"I'm moving to California to study at the Gestalt Therapy Institute, which will train me in additional techniques for dealing with patients' emotions. I know that cancer patients will experience a variety of immobilizing emotions, and I am certain that I can be effective working with them." Again, the staff members were nodding in agreement.

Then I moved to the controversial area. I took a deep breath and said: "Finally, I have a close personal relationship with God and trust that He will guide me on the cancer unit, teaching me what I need to learn and how to comfort the patients, families, and staff." You could have heard a pin drop in the room. Even though St. John's was a Catholic hospital, I was addressing a room full of social workers who, traditionally, did not speak about spiritual matters. After a long silence someone said, "It's great that you have a personal relationship with God, but are you going to be pushing that on the patients and families?"

I smiled and said, "Absolutely not. I don't plan to discuss God unless prompted by a patient or family member. I respect everyone's personal beliefs or lack of belief. My plan is to use God in my own life. I know that working with cancer patients will be challenging and, at times, sad and depressing. I know there will be the possibility of burnout. When I feel overwhelmed with cancer, dying, and loss I will turn to God and let Him guide my actions and fill me with peace and wisdom. That is how I will maintain my stamina and be able to serve the patients, families, and nursing staff."

I'm happy to report that I got the job. God and I moved into the cancer unit. I thought *I* was taking *Him*, but now I know that *He* was taking *me*, for a higher purpose that unfolds in this story.

It was a magical time to be part of the brand new cancer unit at St. John's. The administration was fully behind the project and spared no expense in our training, team building, and funding. A comprehensive team was assembled to manage the needs of the hospital's special cancer patients. On that team were medical oncologists, radiation oncologists, a clinical nurse supervisor, specially trained nurses, an oncology social worker, a pastoral care minister, physical therapists, and an occupational therapist.

During my two years on the cancer unit I learned a lot about cancer and its effects on patients, families, and medical staff. In 1976 the word *cancer* was, in itself, very scary. Personnel from other departments in the hospital were reluctant to come to our unit. We were, after all, the *cancer unit,* located on the top floor of the 6 North tower and filled with all kinds of cancer patients. You could see the fear on people's faces when they got off the elevator. Any visitors or staff from other parts of the hospital sort of held their breath, did whatever they had to do, and hurriedly jumped back onto the elevator.

The popular belief was that a cancer diagnosis was a death sentence, and that maybe cancer was even contagious. People seemed to be afraid to touch the patients. When our patients were picked up and transported to other parts of the hospital for tests or treatment, there was a minimum of physical contact. Family members often told me that friends and neighbors avoided them, for fear they would catch cancer.

On our unit we treated adult patients who had a variety of types of the disease: cancer of the breast, cervix, uterus, throat, lung, brain, bone, bladder, bowel, or pancreas; non-Hodgkin's lymphoma; leukemia; melanoma, and others. At that time the standard treatments were surgery, radiation, and combinations of chemotherapy or the implantation of radioactive isotopes.

By the time patients were admitted to our unit, many of them were already in the end stage of fighting their cancer. They'd spend long periods of time with us or return only sporadically. If their treatments weren't successful there wasn't much hope. Few alternative approaches to cancer treatment were available in hospitals at the time. Dr. Elisabeth Kübler-Ross's landmark book, *On Death and Dying*, with its five stages of death and dying, had recently been published and was being discussed in medical circles.

Meanwhile, patients who responded successfully to surgery, radiation, and/or chemotherapy left our unit and often didn't return. So we didn't get much chance to celebrate the victories—on top of the fact that we were left to deal with many deaths.

From the point of first diagnosis, treatment was pretty doctor-centric: Doctors ordered tests, made diagnoses, and arranged treatments—without much input from the patients or their family members. In those days most patients obediently went along with the doctors' recommendations, afraid to disagree for fear they might make the doctors angry. Patients put their bodies and treatment decisions in the doctors' hands and hoped for the best. Family members asked the doctors questions but often did not understand medical terminology. They also struggled with being in their own state of shock or found that the doctors just didn't have much time for them. Sometimes they were able to discuss their questions with the nursing staff. But generally, family members, too, deferred to the doctors' recommendations.

The bulk of patient care in a hospital is handled by the nursing staff. Nurses are the hands, feet, and heart of a hospital. They take care of the patients' bodies and beds and carry out the doctors' orders, trying to make the patients as comfortable as possible. They dispense medications, oversee baths, change dressings, talk with patients, offer hugs, greet family members, respond to patients' requests, and so much more.

Because I was the first oncology social worker on this brand new unit, my role was not clearly defined. My social service director gave me the luxury of time to just sit and observe the comings and goings of the patients, families, doctors, nurses, and ancillary staff. Fortunately my office was located right next to the lounge and across from the nurses' station and elevator. I was right near all the action. And we had only twenty-some patients, whose rooms were nearby. During this time, I asked God to open my eyes and my other senses and show me how I might be of service.

On our unit, the nurses faced the challenges of controlling patients' symptoms, the many side effects of treatments, and pain, which was often substantial. They had little training in how to deal with the roller coaster of emotions that patients and their family members experienced. They didn't understand why some patients got so angry at them. They didn't know what to do when someone was having an anxiety attack or showing signs of depression. When too many patients died in a short period of time, the nurses became sad and depressed and sometimes burned out. In those cases they might rotate out of the unit for a stint in pediatrics or delivery, just to rebuild their stamina and optimism.

I saw families assembling in patients' rooms or gathering in the lounge or walking the halls, looking lost and overwhelmed. The fatigue, fear, depression, shock, and sadness were written on their faces and embedded in their bodies. Often there were little children or grandparents or extended family and friends who just didn't know what to do with themselves.

Patients were often isolated in their rooms, wanting to talk but finding no one who dared "speak the truth" with them. Family and staff were reluctant to discuss the possibility of death and tended to cover up their emotions. Patients, in turn, picked up on the message to repress their emotions and were thus often silent as well. They either shoved their anxiety, fear, sadness, and depression inside their bodies or erupted with angry outbursts aimed at the nursing staff. Or they became very demanding of special attention, just to have some companionship. Unfortunately the nurses often didn't understand this behavior and would label these patients as "problem patients" to be avoided whenever possible.

Doctors were generally brief in their visits with patients and family members, maintaining what appeared to be an aloof, detached manner. I knew these doctors cared deeply about their patients and had dedicated their careers to fighting cancer. But it didn't show on their faces or in the amount of time they were able to give. Some of this behavior, I realized, was a defense mechanism. After all, these doctors were in the cancer business for the long haul. In a career of twenty or thirty years they couldn't afford to become too emotionally invested in relationships with patients who might die and family members who would leave. These doctors worked long hours and made life-or-death decisions, carrying the weight of the fight against cancer. They were often tired. They had many patients to see in a given day and little time to sit and talk. Moreover, the medical schools that had trained them had done little to prepare them for treating the minds, emotions, and spirits of their patients. But they did the best they could. I observed, too, that when a doctor would let his guard down and attach himself to a particular patient, you would see the devastation on his face if that patient ultimately died. It was difficult to bear.

In this environment, it didn't take long for me to recognize opportunities for my involvement. Here are some of the practices I initiated.

For Patients

I visited patients in their rooms and got to know them on a deep, emotional level. Again, I had the luxury of plenty of time. Sometimes patients would request to speak with me; sometimes I just went in and asked if I could sit down. Given the opportunity, most of them were eager to open up and discuss their fears, hopes, frustrations, and bewilderment, not to mention their problems dealing with their family members and their fear of dying. Usually these discussions did not occur on the first visit but instead blossomed gradually over a period of time—and with the establishment of trust.

As I developed close personal relationships with many of the patients, I noticed some relief in their physical symptoms of pain or depression or anxiety. I also saw increased optimism, improved relationships with their family members, and more willingness to participate in their own healing. They were eager to learn what they could do to fight the cancer. I engaged them in art therapy, which gave them the opportunity to explore their deepest feelings. I led them through deep-relaxation exercises, which allowed their bodies to let go of fear and tension. And I taught them visualization techniques, which improved the functioning of their immune systems and strengthened their bodies as well as their psyches.

With every new patient I would ask a straightforward, yet profound question: "Are you ready to die? You are at a fork in the road and you have to make a decision. Do you want to give up or do you want to fight?" Yes, this approach was risky. But it was also necessary. I wanted to teach patients that they had power either way: If they were at the end stage of their disease, it was okay for them to let go, to surrender to death; I could help them with that journey. If they were depressed, I could help them regain a sense of strength and teach them what they could do to fight the cancer. If they were too immobilized to take any action, I could help them regain their inner strength and then make a clear decision. If they wanted to change their treatment plan, I could arrange a meeting with their doctor. If they wanted to be discharged and die at home, I could work with them and their families to set up in-home hospice or assistance care.

The important factor was to involve the patient in the decision-making process and ensure his or her quality of life. When patients were dying I helped them put their affairs in order, mend their relationships with family, say goodbye, and prepare for their spiritual journey into the next dimension. In many cases I was at the bedside when a patient passed on, and I felt blessed and honored to be present. Some patients, conversely, did not want any help at all, and I respected their decisions. Whatever their needs and choices, each patient taught me so much about cancer and dignity.

For Family Members

I met with family members at their request, at the suggestion of the nursing staff, or by simply randomly introducing myself and asking if I could be of some assistance. Many family members were afraid to reveal their own feelings and needs to their patients out of a sense of protection. By neglecting those needs, they often built up resentment or felt guilty when they took time for themselves. I encouraged them to speak from their hearts and discuss their true emotions with their patients. I reassured them that their openness would, in turn, encourage their patients to open up too—to everyone's benefit. Gradually these families began talking on a real level of honesty and were able to work together to solve the day-to-day challenges of living with cancer. Whenever this transformation occurred I saw a reduction in tension and an increase in joy in the moment, laughter, and cohesion. I saw families crying, embracing, kissing, hugging, making plans together.

I coached families on how to prepare for their visits with doctors: "Write your questions down beforehand. Ask the doctor to sit down for a minute so that you can talk to him. Don't be afraid or embarrassed to say you don't understand a procedure or a medication. There are no dumb questions. Don't be afraid to say you disagree with the doctor's recommendation. Take your power, for you and your patient."

I organized a weekly group for families of patients who had been newly diagnosed, who were currently on the unit, who had been discharged, or who had died. It was a very popular group. It became a safe place for family members to express their myriad emotions, without fear of burdening their patients. Group gave family members the chance to discuss their fears, fatigue, anger, depression, hopes, shock, feelings of being overwhelmed; their guilt, their desire to run away, their struggles—with people who could understand because they were going through the same thing. Many long-term friendships were established in the group, and many people stayed in the group for years as core members. Family members who participated in the group were less likely to become sick themselves and had a better re-entry into life if their patient died. Children whose parents attended the group had a better chance of receiving the individual attention and guidance they so desperately needed, thanks to the support and guidance the group offered.

For the Nurses

The nurses' need for emotional support was plain to see. The cancer unit was a tough place to work. Cancer is a very challenging disease. At the worst it can kill people. At the least, treatments to save peoples' lives can take a huge toll on their bodies, minds, spirits, and emotions. Surgical incisions, the loss of organs and body parts, hair loss, weight loss, incontinence, the loss of appetite, nausea and diarrhea from chemotherapy and radiation, the roller coaster of emotions—the list of challenges is long and seemingly unending at times.

The nurses were on the front lines for all of this each day. They were responsible not only for patient care and inter-actions with family members, but also their *own* emotional, psychological, and physical reactions to dealing with cancer and loss. So for them I organized a weekly support group, which met off premises whenever possible. It was important for us to get away from the hospital; to be in an atmosphere that was intimate and uplifting—that would promote sharing and healing. We often met in my home or sometimes at the beach. I also taught the nurses about the psychological and emotional needs of patients and their families, and offered individual counseling and supportive hugs. We actually supported each other. We laughed and cried and talked with each other, which boosted morale on the unit. We had potluck lunches and took time to relax and play together. I can't say enough good things about our nurses. They were angels who truly loved the patients and invested deeply in them. And they showed their feelings with hugs and kisses and tears.

For Myself

Working on the cancer unit was extremely rewarding, yet challenging too. I learned so much from the patients and their family members, and I found it a privilege to share their journeys with cancer. From the doctors, the nurses, the ancillary staff, and the social service department I gained considerable knowledge about the various types of cancer and their treatment options, along with insights on the complex workings of a hospital.

Like the other staff members, I was often tired from the weight of the responsibility. Fighting cancer is a war, and it takes a lot out of you. So, true to my original word, when I felt overwhelmed I would turn to God and ask for assistance, guidance, and sustenance. Without fail God would give me what I needed: insight into a problem followed by a viable solution; an intervention for a patient or a family member; the release of my anxiety, fear, or depression; the return of a state of peacefulness in my body; a scripture to inspire my spirit. Indeed, on many occasions I had the pleasure of engaging in spiritual discussions and prayer with patients, family members, and staff.

I learned many powerful lessons working on the cancer unit. Most important among them:

+ Truly live in the moment and celebrate each day as if it were your last.

+ Be humble and gentle with yourself in moments of weakness and despair.

+ Take deliberate, proactive care of your body, mind, emotions, and spirit to diminish the possibility of developing a life-threatening illness.

+ You're going to die someday, so keep your affairs in order: Don't take your relationships for granted. Don't assume that you have an infinite amount of time. Be sure to tell people that you love them. Work on solving problems and conflicts. Move toward forgiveness and reconciliation. With respect to your finances, designate a beneficiary on your checking and savings accounts; establish a will and a trust. For the care of your own body, in case you become incapacitated, establish an advanced medical directive that includes a living will and a durable power of attorney for health care. Let your family know if you want a burial or a cremation when you die.

+ Be courageous in your aspirations. You have nothing to lose. Within the finite amount of time you have on earth, dare to dream and set specific goals for yourself. Believe that you are worthy of achieving the desires of your heart, and then work hard, with single-minded focus, to achieve each goal. If you meet with resistance or temporary failure, don't be discouraged and don't lose hope. Learn from mistakes, come up with a better plan or strategy, and move forward. Don't be afraid to risk.

+ Share life's journey with people and animals you love.

+ It takes teamwork to win the war against cancer.

+ The gift of life is a blessing, fraught with opportunities for personal growth and spiritual insight. Share what you have learned, and learn from others as well.

+ Do not fear death. Your spirit continues in the next dimension.

+ God is always with you and will help you with all things.

In 1978 I left St. John's and opened my own private practice in cancer counseling and psychotherapy. I was eager to collaborate with patients who had recently been diagnosed with cancer, believing that our work together could increase their chances of survival. I was motivated by the training I had done with Dr O. Carl Simonton and Stephanie Matthews-Simonton of the Cancer Counseling and Research Center in Fort Worth, Texas. They believed that all people have cancer cells in their bodies, monitored and controlled by their immune systems. The Simontons developed the theory that six to eighteen months prior to the development of a tumor, many cancer patients have incurred some kind of trauma or loss. The stress of that event and whether or not they have fully worked through their emotional reactions might cause their immune systems to become depressed and allow the cancer cells to multiply and proliferate. These groundbreaking theories were originally published in the Simontons' *Cancer Self-Help Education* workbook. The Simontons later released their bestselling classic, *Getting Well Again: A Step-by-Step, Self-Help Guide to Overcoming Cancer for Patients and Their Families*.

The Simontons' theory did not blame cancer patients as though they had somehow created their own cancer. Instead it presented the hopeful, revolutionary idea that cancer patients could learn how to turn their cancer around by making changes in their lives. The Simontons initiated the use of art therapy, guided meditation, and cancer counseling workbooks to empower cancer patients to release negative emotions, build positive expectations, and boost the functioning of the immune system. The Simontons believed in the mind-body-emotions connection. Using their techniques with end-stage cancer patients, they were able to document increases in both lifespan and quality of life, as well as a reduction in patients' pain.

If the Simontons could get these kinds of results with end-stage cancer patients, just imagine what I could achieve with patients who had only recently been diagnosed! My plan was to combine the Simontons' techniques with individual long-term psychotherapy. The key was to *engage patients in the fight for their lives,* from the beginning of treatment. No more just putting the responsibility in the doctors' hands.

In my cancer counseling sessions, patients and I could evaluate all areas of their lives, including their past priorities, and restructure what wasn't working. We could concentrate on creating health and eliminating fear. We could change diet, incorporate exercise, add relaxation and meditation techniques, and structure time for relaxation. We could alleviate anxiety and depression. We could use dream analysis to explore deeper issues in the unconscious. We could identify areas of the patients' lives where they were holding resentment or anger and work toward forgiveness. We could tap into the power of prayer. We could build teamwork with patients' family members.

I thought that the key to the success of my practice would be to get referrals from doctors. So I approached the medical oncologists I had been working with and told them of my plans. I expressed my enthusiasm and optimism. I gave them my business cards, announcements, and brochures. I pitched working in conjunction with their practices. I did the same with other doctors in the area. I made follow-up calls and dropped into their offices. I waited. And waited. And waited.

I'm sad to report that I never got even one referral from any doctor. I was especially disappointed in the group of medical oncologists who had been my colleagues at St. John's. They were intimately aware of the scope of my work. We had collaborated side by side in the cancer unit for two years. They had seen me with patients and their families, and they'd read the detailed descriptions and rec-ommendations I had written in each patient's chart. But apparently they didn't believe in the idea of cancer coun-seling or empowering patients and their family members. For them, it seemed, it was enough to treat the body alone. It was 1978, after all, and most mainstream doctors were simply not ready to embrace a more comprehensive approach to dealing with cancer patients.

The bulk of the clients I did have came from word of mouth. I worked with them in their homes. I followed through with my initial plans and added more techniques as we went along. As I learned and my clients and their families benefited from the work we were doing together, I wrote and presented professional papers in Los Angeles.

It was a wonderful period in my life. The people and the work touched my heart and would ultimately influence my work with other types of clients throughout my career.

From that time forward I became a holistic psychotherapist, treating the bodies, minds, emotions, and spirits of my clients.

Over the last thirty-five years I have had the honor to treat hundreds of men, women, and adolescents facing a variety of life challenges: chronic and life-threatening illness; debilitating depression and anxiety; homelessness; alcohol, food, or drug addictions; childhood abuse and neglect; the death of a family member; post-traumatic stress; hearts broken from a failed relationship or divorce; codependency; the loss of employment; excessive debt; marital discord; troubled family relationships. To each of my clients I have brought the perspective of the body-mind-emotions-spirit connection.

I have found that when people are willing to do the work in therapy and take responsibility for their own lives, they are able to achieve health, healing, and transformation. What do I mean by "do the work" in therapy and "achieve health"? In order to transform your life, you must begin with a picture of what you don't like about your current life and what you hope to achieve in therapy. Then you must make a commitment of time, personal effort, willingness to learn and explore all the parts of yourself—conscious and unconscious—as well as an openness to change old habits, coping skills, and attitudes that are self-defeating. This process is slow, demanding, frightening at times, but ultimately empowering and liberating. The therapist is your guide, but you must do the work on yourself.

Similarly, good health is a state of being in your body that requires time, commitment, consistency, and daily effort to achieve. Diet; exercise; peaceful connection with mind, emotions, and spirit; regular medical checkups; attention to physical symptoms before they develop into serious illnesses; achieving balance in your life—they all require work.

I've been amazed by the resiliency of the human spirit as well as the body and brain's capacity for healing and rejuvenation. And I have continued to incorporate God into my work, witnessing in the process how the Spirit really works in peoples' lives—with a power far greater than our own.

To expand my knowledge about the body-mind-emotions-spirit connection, I trained and studied at the Jin Shin Do Acupressure Foundation and the C.G. Jung Institute and library in Los Angeles. Additionally, I studied Hatha yoga, and I have maintained a yoga practice for the last twenty years under the loving guidance of Riayn Shumacher. In 2010 I released my first book, *Creating A Healthy Life and Marriage: A Holistic Approach: Body, Mind, Emotions and Spirit*. The book germinated inside me for fifteen years and was written in stages, according to the clinical and personal lessons that I learned. The book reflects my treatment philosophy that each of us can be healed of the emotional, psychological, physical, and spiritual wounds from child-hood and adulthood by the grace and faithfulness of God's assistance, and through learning healthy coping skills that will bring us an intimate relationship with our *Self* and others. In the book, I share stories of my personal healing and transformation, along with those of my clients.

Prologue

IN NOVEMBER 2011 MY HUSBAND WAS DIAGNOSED WITH A very aggressive form of prostate cancer. We aren't talking about a low-risk, "active surveillance" type of prostate cancer or even a moderate-risk, radiation-only type, but a dangerous, life-threatening type of prostate cancer. The moment we learned the seriousness of his diagnosis, it was as if we had been shot into the air by a cannon. We were hurtling helplessly through space, not knowing where we would land or what we should do, all the while sensing that our lives would never again be the same. In the days that followed, we had to land on our feet and learn to navigate the new terrain. We had to make strategic decisions quickly. We had no time to lose.

When I left St. John's Hospital in 1978, all those years ago, I never imagined I would one day return as the wife of a man diagnosed with prostate cancer.

This is a book I never wanted to write.

It's difficult for me for several reasons. For starters, I was 48 years old when I met my husband and 49 when we got married. We've now been married for twenty years. Before I met my husband my life had been very difficult—pretty sad and lonely, in fact. I had been searching for him my whole life. So the possibility of losing him to prostate cancer was—and still is—terrifying. This book was also hard for me to write because when I first began doing so, it was only six months after my husband's diagnosis and I was still pretty raw. Moreover, I had no idea how our story would unfold.

I chose to go ahead and write, however, because I knew it would be healing for me. As importantly, I believed that my experiences would be helpful to other people who are walking a similar path. I wish there was no audience for this book, but I know that there are millions of men around the world who are diagnosed with prostate cancer. The cancer affects them *and* the people who love them.

What I want to present in this book is a full firsthand picture of the emotional and psychological toll that prostate cancer has on patients and their loved ones. I want to show how it affects them on the *inside*; the parts that may be invisible to others but are very real: the mind, emotions, and spirit. It is my firm belief that understanding and treating these dimensions of the disease as well as the body, **in a holistic approach,** can lead to a better prognosis for the prostate cancer patient—and that it can also prevent family caretakers from developing their own medical problems due to stress.

Over the two-year period I've been writing this book, I have gained painful yet valuable insight into the whole dynamics of cancer, treatment, and healing. This insight is so much more real and organic than the theories I employed as an oncology social worker back in the 1970s. In those days my knowledge was *only* theoretical, or limited to what I gleaned or intuited from my work with patients, family members, and the medical staff. I had only a vague idea what the patients and their family members were going through. I didn't truly understand the deep impact of having a family member living with cancer. So my counsel to patients and their families, while well intended, was undoubtedly a bit superficial.

In this book I want to earnestly and honestly share the experiences my husband and I have had with prostate cancer so far, in hopes that you will find comfort and power from the shared experiences whether you're the patient or the patient's loved one. You will find here practical suggestions for navigating the medical system, insight into your own emotional-psychological-spiritual processes, strategies for battling prostate cancer in particular, and the courage to fight prostate cancer with all your might—while maintaining a loving relationship. I pray that by reading our story, you will be blessed in some way and that *you will find your Inner Warrior* (a person who is strong in body, mind, emotions, and spirit; a person with fierce determination to live, who is disciplined and well armed for the battle with cancer)—again, whether you're the patient or the patient's loved one.

I believe that your spirit is your strongest personal weapon. Because I use the term "spirit" throughout this book, I would like to share a passage (pages 93-94) from *Creating A Healthy Life and Marriage* that explains this concept:

> "Your spirit is that part of you which is individual and unique, which has tremendous power, which is designed to guide you in the process of actualizing your divine destiny.
>
> Your spirit is the most transcendent part of you. It does not age or decay, it does not die, and it always seeks your highest good. It often knows what you should do before your mind, emotions, and body have figured it out. Your spirit may have been cramped, battered, or abused by your family of origin, but it cannot be extinguished, even in death. It is the best and most permanent part of you. It is the strongest part of you.
>
> Your spirit can help heal you of your wounds, however severe they may be. It seeks to connect you with your Higher Power but will always give you the right not to. Your spirit will speak to you in dreams, in writing, in art, in dance, in nature, in animals.
>
> When you are quiet, when you make time to listen, it will speak to you in a quiet inner voice. The emerging voice of the spirit does not have ... negative characteristics. ... Your spiritual voice will give you only messages of love, approval, encouragement, hope, inspiration, creation, and forgiveness. It will caution you to avoid danger and wrongdoing. It will

confront you when you have done wrong and call you to make amends.

The Creator has given you all the tools for a happy, healthy life and relationships. Everything you need is within you. You have only to look."

One final note before we begin: Although I'm writing specifically about prostate cancer, I'm confident that the principles I present here apply to men and women with any form of cancer—as well as their family members.

CHAPTER ONE

The Shock of the Diagnosis

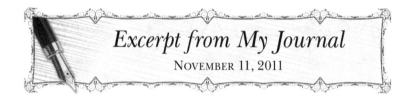

Excerpt from My Journal
NOVEMBER 11, 2011

A DATE THAT OCCURS ONLY ONCE IN A LIFETIME. MY HUSBAND and I were at home at 5:30 p.m. on a Friday night, waiting for a call from his urologist. The day before, my husband had gone into the hospital to get a biopsy of his prostate. His latest PSA reading was a 6 and the doctor had felt a firmness on the right side of the prostate, which had never been present on any previous digital exam.

My husband's PSA had been fluctuating between 4 and 6 for the last two years, and the urologist had been monitoring him closely. Taking a biopsy had been discussed as a possibility, but the doctor never firmly recommended it before, and my husband was a little afraid of the procedure. The risks of fever and infection seemed greater than the need for the biopsy, so it was decided to take a PSA test and undergo a digital exam every three months while following the doctor's protocol for what he believed was an "anti-inflammatory diet" that restricted caffeine, chocolate, alcohol, and spicy food.

I had been a little nervous to hear the results of the biopsy, but I didn't want to say anything about it to my husband for fear of making him more nervous. He told me later that he had a recurring feeling of dread throughout the day that we were going to hear something bad.

When the phone rang and we put on the speaker, there was a heavy tone in the doctor's voice. He said, "I am very sorry but I have some news that isn't good. The Gleason score from the biopsy is 9 (4+5). There is cancer in the prostate that is very aggressive. It is on the right side of the prostate and there is some on the left side. We don't yet know the percentage of cancer in the six core samples, which will be on the pathology report. I will set aside forty-five minutes on Tuesday to meet with both of you, and we will discuss the alternatives for treatment. In the meantime, do your own research on the Internet."

On the other end of the line, my husband and I both said at the same time, "9? How could it be a 9?" We both thought, "You're kidding, right? You must have called us with someone else's biopsy results."

We were both in shock, and it was hard to hear or concentrate on what the doctor was saying. We were expecting no cancer at all or a Gleason score of 6. Nine was unexpected, alarming, and frightening. We were both immediately overwhelmed, and our bodies and our brains were shutting down.

We struggled to regain some control and began asking questions:

- *What exactly does the Gleason score mean?*
- *How could it be so high?*
- *How could the cancer be so advanced when firmness was never detected in the previous digital exams?*
- *How could the Gleason score be so high when the PSA number was low?*
- *How long could the cancer have been there?*

Questions, shock, fear, dread, and terror ran through our minds and bodies.

It was now 6:15 p.m. on a Friday night, and we weren't going to see the doctor for four full days. What were we supposed to do? We stared at each other with wide eyes and felt like someone had kicked us in the stomach. We were speechless....

No one is ever prepared to hear that they, or someone they love, have cancer. Even today in our modern age, *cancer* is still a scary word. It implies the possibility of death and loss, and it strikes fear in our very core.

Our bodies react to the news with an immediate, automatic response. Our pupils dilate so that we can see more clearly. Our hearts beat faster and pump blood through vessels that have become constricted, so that our bodies get extra nourishment. Our brains give the signal to release into our systems large amounts of adrenaline and the stress hormone cortisol, to give us extra strength. Our breathing becomes rapid and shallow as we are poised to take action.

This reaction from the sympathetic nervous system gives us a high dose of energy so that, faced with the danger, we can make a quick decision to fight or flee—the so-called *fight/flight response*. Once we make a decision and take action, our bodies return to a state of rest. Our heart rate slows down, our pupils return to normal size, we relax, and adrenaline and cortisol stop being released.

Brain researchers have recently discovered that there is a third possible reaction to danger: *immobilization*. In this response the body has the same sympathetic nervous system reactions and is filled with the same high dose of energy, adrenaline, and cortisol. But the person has a frozen, "deer caught in the headlights of a car" reaction. He neither fights nor flees but instead remains caught in this heightened arousal state, immobilized by fear. As such, his heart does not return to a resting rate, the adrenaline and cortisol continue to course through his veins, and his breathing remains rapid and shallow. His brain is unable to make a decision and remains on high alert. His legs do not carry him to safety, his body remains tense, and he does not escape the danger or the fear. This is a very unhealthy and exhausting response that, over time, will depress the functioning of his immune system and lock his psyche into a panic state.

All people are different and have their own characteristic responses to danger. Some of us are fighters, some people run away, some become immobilized. Or we may respond to the danger in all three ways.

The problem with cancer in particular is that it is not just an immediate danger that you can fight or run from and then the danger is over. Cancer is an ever-present, life-threatening danger with an indefinite timeline. Cancer threatens the person with the diagnosis and his/her family as well. So from the point of first diagnosis, living with cancer puts our bodies, minds, emotions, and spirits in a state of high alert and shock.

My husband and I responded to his diagnosis very differently. He was temporarily immobilized. I sprang into action, even though I was still in shock. I told my husband, "I'm going to call Silent Unity and have them pray for us." (Silent Unity—*www.silentunity.org*—is a non-denominational spiritual organization with a healing ministry, dedicated to providing free affirmative prayer for people around the world twenty-four hours a day, seven days a week. The organization receives more than 3,700 calls a day. U.S.: (800) 669-7729; International: (01) (816) 969-2000. Silent Unity's monthly book of daily meditations is called *Daily Word*). I dialed the 800 number, put on the speaker, and told the prayer minister about the prostate cancer and the high Gleason score. I asked her to pray for both of us.

From that point on I can honestly say that we don't remember what the woman said. But her voice was soft, soothing, and comforting. We sat there, holding each other. I don't believe we cried; we were too scared. Throughout my life I have called Silent Unity during times of crisis. It was an automatic response from my spirit.

Next, I suggested to my husband that he call his first cousin and tell him the news, as his cousin had been diagnosed with prostate cancer two years previously and had chosen to be treated with proton radiation therapy at Loma Linda Medical Center. My husband picked up the phone and called his cousin, who was very sorry to hear the news and was gracious enough to spend forty-five minutes describing his own experience. His biopsy results had shown a Gleason score of 6, and he had chosen to have proton radiation as his sole treatment, five days a week for nine weeks. While my husband and his cousin were talking, I could see that my husband was regaining control of his body. His voice was getting stronger, his breathing was relaxing a bit, and he was freed to ask his cousin a series of questions. When he finished the call he said he felt calmer.

I then suggested that he might want to call his older brother, who has always been a source of support and reason. When he made that call, delivered the news, and heard his brother's voice, I could see that, once again, he became calmer. He was sharing the burden and receiving love and encouragement. His brother was shocked and gave us as much comfort as he could muster in the moment. We made plans to have breakfast with him two days later, on Sunday.

With each of these phone calls I, too, began to relax and breathe a little easier. At this point I asked my husband if I could call my son. I wanted to share the news with him, and I also wanted to get the email address of my ex-husband, who had been battling prostate cancer for eight years. I wanted to ask him if he would give us a consultation.

My husband told me it was okay to make the call to my son, and that I could also call my daughter and brother. But he didn't want to tell anyone else except for his two daughters and his ex-wife. "Only immediate family," he said. "I don't want people to feel sorry for me. I don't want them to look at me differently now that I have cancer. I'm the same person I was before I got the diagnosis." I was glad he was making decisions, retaking control of his life. He was no longer immobilized.

I called my son and told him I wanted his father's email address. He asked why, knowing we were getting the biopsy results that day. I told him the news was bad and that we wanted to ask his dad some questions about the treatment of his prostate cancer. I was crying and I could barely talk.

My son told me he loved us, that he and his wife would pray for us, and that he would get me the email address of his father. When I got the address later that night I wrote a quick note, telling my ex-husband the diagnosis and asking if we might be able to arrange a phone consultation that weekend. I was too exhausted to call anyone else.

After that phone call, I sat down with my husband and said to him: "We are One Body, with Four Legs. I am going to be with you every step of the way." Then we wrapped our arms around each other and cried.

Neither one of us had any appetite, but we knew we should eat something. So we struggled to eat a bowl of soup, then suddenly felt the weight of our exhaustion. I think the shock set in again. We tumbled into bed and held tightly to one another. My husband said, "We are the same people today that we were yesterday," and then we fell asleep. I prayed for my husband throughout the night. I literally put my hand on him and prayed over and over, with all my might: "Please, please, please God, heal my husband of this cancer."

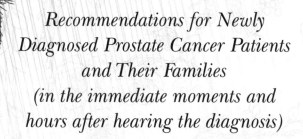

*Recommendations for Newly
Diagnosed Prostate Cancer Patients
and Their Families
(in the immediate moments and
hours after hearing the diagnosis)*

1. Be aware that you will be in shock, and know that this is normal. Shock is a temporary mechanism that prevents you from being overwhelmed. You may be unable to speak, and you may not remember what people say to you. Your body may shut down, and you may be unable to walk or stand. Your brain may become fuzzy.

2. To recover from the shock, try to mobilize yourselves by taking some sort of action.

3. Talk with each other and decide who you will tell about the diagnosis.

4. Make some strategic phone calls to people who can offer you support, prayers, encouragement, and hope. Hearing their voices and feeling their love will calm you down and give you courage. You need the support, and you'll benefit from it.

5. Be gentle with your body and understand that you will experience fatigue, nausea, digestive disturbances, and mental confusion.

6. Consider asking God to help you. Some studies show that people who pray and are prayed for have fewer complications, lower overall adverse outcomes, lower levels of negative emotions, higher levels of health self-efficacy, higher levels of functional well-being, more likeliness to find blessings in their lives, and less fear of death.

www.cancer.org/treatment/treatments andsideeffects/complementaryand alternativemedicine/mindbodyandspirit/ spirituality-and-prayer

www.ncbi.nlm.nih.gov/pubmed/22894887

archinte.jamanetwork.com/article.aspx? articleid=485161

onlinelibrary.wiley.com/doi/10.1002/ pon.1129/abstract

7. Accept the love and support that people want to give you. It's a two-way blessing: you are blessed by their gift, and you bless them by giving them the opportunity to help you. Don't try to fight cancer all by yourself.

8. Hug and hold each other; it will comfort you.

9. Don't be afraid to cry. It is not a sign of weakness. The tears will release stress and cleanse your spirit.

10. Try to get some sleep, which will replenish your energy and help your immune system during the cancer fight.

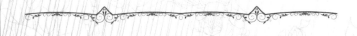

CHAPTER TWO

Facing Our Immediate Fears

ONCE THE SHOCK OF THE PROSTATE CANCER DIAGNOSIS wears off a bit, we enter into the stage of *fear*. According to my husband, here are the key fears of the man who has been diagnosed:

+ Am I going to die, and will the cancer ravage my body?
+ Will the treatments designed to save my life cause a loss of sexual function and/or incontinence?
+ Can I get through this?
+ Are people going to treat me differently?

The main fears for the family members and other loved ones, meanwhile:

+ Is my husband (father/brother/friend/etc.) going to suffer, and will he die?
+ Did I do something to cause the cancer?

+ Will I be able to survive this?
+ How will we get through this?

In my case, the fears didn't set in until after I had gone to bed that fateful Friday night and lay awake in the darkness. A series of thoughts and questions flooded my mind: "Is my husband going to die?" "How will I live if he dies?" "If he dies, then I want to die too. I couldn't stand to live life without him." These fears ran through my head throughout the night. I have found that I am always more vulnerable to fear at night, when it is dark. The more fears that surfaced that long night, the more frightened I became. I struggled to sleep. My body was filled with stress and anxiety.

Although my husband and I had promised each other that we would talk about all of our feelings, the thoughts in my head were too depressing and too scary to share with him. I didn't want to frighten or depress him, so I kept my fears to myself—and they continued to haunt and terrorize me. I suspect my husband had similar fears running through his head that he, too, kept to himself.

I decided that **my journal** would be a safe place for me to release and explore all of my feelings, and that it would give me a way to comfort myself. I knew I didn't have too many other options. Once I told my children what was going on, I knew they would have their own sets of fears and that they would be looking for me to be their source of strength. Moreover, because my husband wanted to keep the news strictly in the immediate family, I wouldn't be able to talk to any neighbors or friends about it.

I have been journaling for more than thirty years, so this coping strategy was entirely natural for me. In my journal I confide in God and ask Him to guide and comfort me. I express my darkest emotions and feelings of despair, panic, depression, and helplessness. As I write, my body is able to relax and release the tension. Sometimes I cry, sometimes I cuss, sometimes I express my anger in **BIG BOLD LETTERS**, sometimes I request a scripture to guide me, sometimes I pray. In the process of writing I connect with my heart, my body, my emotions, my mind, and my spirit. Through journaling I find wholeness and strength, inspiration and guidance. I am released from the *fight/flight/immobilization* response.

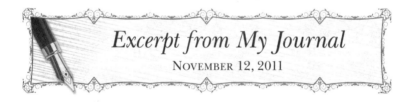

Excerpt from My Journal
NOVEMBER 12, 2011

WHEN WE WOKE UP, WE LAY IN BED A LONG WHILE AND TALKED. We expressed our shock, our confusion about what was happening, our concerns about which treatment we would select, our ignorance about prostate cancer, how our bodies were reacting to the stress. It was good for both of us to talk and bond together. We were choosing to face this challenge together, as partners. I told my husband we could write a book about our

*journey with cancer, and he said, "Only if the outcome is good."
I said that sharing our experience might help other people.*

*When we got up, I went to my computer to do some research
about prostate cancer. I knew that gathering information and
educating myself would be a healthy way to combat my fears.
In terms of understanding my own coping mechanisms, I know
that if I engage my brain when facing an emergency, my emotions and body will calm down and my spirit will guide me
in the right direction.*

*When I worked at St. John's Hospital, I never knowingly
worked with any man who had prostate cancer. I knew nothing about it. In hindsight, I may have worked with men whose
primary prostate cancer had metastasized to other parts of their
bodies. I also didn't understand what "Gleason score of 9
(4+5)" meant. For all I knew it might be terrible and my husband might be on the verge of dying that very day. I knew that
"knowledge is power," so I wanted to educate myself and see
just how bad this diagnosis was and what we might be able to
do about it.*

*I didn't know exactly where to start, so I Googled "Prostate can-
cer, Gleason score of 9." I checked out the various links and
began to amass a lot of preliminary information about prostate
cancer. One especially helpful site was: Prostate Cancer Research
Institute (PCRI), www.prostate-cancer.org; Helpline: (800)
641-7274. On that site there are tabs for many topics, like:
"What Is Prostate Cancer?" "Causes," "Signs and Symptoms,"
"Stages," "Grades," "Treatments," "Side Effects," "Prognosis,"*

"Recurrence," "Types," "Open Discussion Forums," "Clinical Trials," "Multimedia Teaching Aids," "Videos to Empower You," as well as links to other sites.

I learned that Gleason scores reveal the relative risk of prostate cancer, with Gleason 6, mild risk; Gleason 7-8, moderate risk; Gleason 9-10, very high risk. When I read that I became even more scared. My husband had a biopsy Gleason score of 9. My fears were diminished, however, when I read that there are many new treatment methods for treating even advanced cases of prostate cancer. Having a Gleason score of 9 is not necessarily a death sentence. That gave me some hope and courage.

*I printed out each article I read, for future reference and to share with my husband. In addition, I developed an outline—entitled **PROSTATE CANCER PROFILE**—that contained topics I wanted to discuss in our Tuesday meeting with the urologist. I made three copies: one for my husband, one for me, and one for the doctor. I knew the outline would keep us on track during the discussion, when our emotions might easily overtake us. I didn't understand many of the terms, but I was sure the doctor could educate us.*

PROSTATE CANCER PROFILE

MOST RECENT PSA

GLEASON SCORE

6 or less: *called "well differentiated or low-grade"*
7: *called "moderately differentiated or intermediate-grade"*
8-10: *called "poorly differentiated or high-grade"*
Right lobe:
Left lobe:

PERCENTAGE OF CORE BIOPSIES POSITIVE FOR CANCER

Right lobe:
Left lobe:

TYPE OF CANCER

Right lobe:
Left lobe:

DIAGNOSTIC TESTS WE MAY REQUEST

1. *TRANSRECTAL ULTRASOUND*
2. *SERUM PAP*
3. *CT SCAN OF INTERNAL ORGANS*
4. *MRI SPECTROSCOPY*
5. *BONE SCAN*

TREATMENT CHOICES

1. *ACTIVE SURVEILLANCE*
2. *RADICAL PROSTATECTOMY—TRADITIONAL*
3. *ROBOTIC-ASSISTED RADICAL PROSTATECTOMY WITH PRESERVATION OF ERECTILE NERVES*
4. *EXTERNAL BEAM RADIATION*
5. *EXTERNAL BEAM RADIATION 3D CONFORMAL*
6. *PROTON THERAPY (LOMA LINDA)*
7. *HORMONE THERAPY*
8. *ANALOGS OF LH-RH*
9. *ANTIANDROGENS*
10. *CHEMICAL CASTRATION VIA ZOLADEX*
11. *SINGLE VS. COMBINED THERAPY*

CLINICAL STAGING PARTIN TABLES
(PSA LEVEL, GLEASON GRADE, CLINICAL STAGE)

1. *COMPLETELY ORGAN-CONFINED*
2. *ESTABLISHED CAPSULAR PENETRATION*
3. *EXTENSION INTO SEMINAL VESICLES*
4. *SPREAD TO LYMPH NODES*

I gathered as much information as I could before becoming completely overwhelmed. I didn't understand any of it. There was so much to read and learn. This was such a sharp learning curve, and my brain was not functioning very well.

I have to say that we are blessed to be living in the age of computers and the Internet. We have access to the Internet twenty-four hours a day. When we are alone and frightened we can turn on the lights, turn off our fears, turn on the computer. Gathering information, educating yourself, and reading about treatment options are excellent ways to mobilize your strength, your sense of fighting the cancer.

I showed the printouts to my husband. He was grateful that I was taking the lead and providing some initial education for us. We were in a rush that morning as we had tickets to a college football game that afternoon. We decided to go to the game, thinking it might be a good distraction for us.

Our movements that day were lethargic. We ate a bit, dressed, drove to the game, walked to our seats, but we were both very mechanical and slow. We were still in a daze. As we watched the game and interacted a bit with our seatmates, I wondered to myself, with tears streaming down my cheeks (which were turned away from my husband): "Is this the last game we will see together?"

Fortunately it turned out to be what I call a "state of grace" day. That's the kind of day when God gives you a blessing all day long; things turn out perfectly, with no effort. I have long ago learned to embrace this kind of day. Our team managed to win the game. The people sitting all around us were friendly, fun, and easy to interact with. The weather was perfect. The sights and sounds of the marching band, the jets flying overhead, and the salute to our veterans filled our spirits with temporary joy and relaxation. It was good for us to stand up, shout, and cheer on our team. It was fun connecting with other people. For these three hours we forgot about the cancer. Despite all of these benefits, however, I could not manage to eat even one bite of my popcorn, which is one of my favorite foods.

When we got home we were exhausted once again, and we returned to our state of shock. I had to push myself to make the remaining phone calls to family. I phoned my daughter, who was quite upset to hear the news. She said she and her husband would begin praying for us daily and that she would do serious research on the subject for us.

Next I called my brother, who lives out of state. I told him the news and then broke down, crying, "I don't want to lose him." He said, "Of course you don't, and we don't want to lose him either. He is one of the sweetest men in the world. We will pray for you, and we love you."

We couldn't eat much dinner, although we had barely eaten the whole day. Our stomachs were upset, and we both had diarrhea. We tried to watch some television but we couldn't really concentrate. We tumbled into bed early.

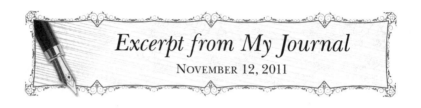

Excerpt from My Journal
November 12, 2011

*This is a new chapter in our marriage of nineteen years.
We have shared the deaths of family members, loss of jobs, problems with our children, medical problems, fluctuating incomes,
growing careers, and deep love for one another.*

*This is a new beginning. The start of something new. Our
wakeup call to cherish each and every day. Our second honeymoon. Our journey into the unknown.*

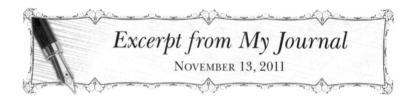

Excerpt from My Journal
November 13, 2011

*This morning we had breakfast with my husband's
brother. Over the years, we have comforted each other through
a variety of situations, and this day was no exception. As we
sat at the deli, each of us looked tense, and worry about the
cancer was a heavy cloud over us. We talked about our shock,
our fears about what lay ahead, about the unknown. It was a
pretty grave meeting. The love amongst us, however, was
stronger than the fear, so we knew being together was a good
thing. Of course my brother-in-law also worried about him-*

self: Was he, too, going to develop prostate cancer? The brothers seemed to recall that their father had some problem with his prostate, though they did not know the specifics.

When we got home we called my ex-husband, who was most gracious to share his own eight-year history with prostate cancer. He had already experienced surgery, radiation, and hormone treatments, and he encouraged my husband to take the most aggressive approach to killing the cancer. He said that the side effects were tolerable and not to be feared. This phone call and discussion were invaluable to my husband. It gave him the opportunity to discuss his fears, gain knowledge about treatment options, and receive encouragement and wisdom from a man who had walked the same path. It also pointed him in the direction of having a radical prostatectomy, though he still clung to the desire to have only radiation therapy. Over the ensuing months we had many similar phone discussions, which were always a blessing to us.

In the afternoon we took a nap, then watched movies with our puppy. We both had little to no appetite at dinner time and went to bed early.

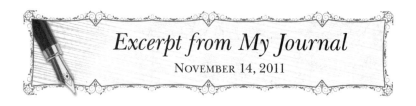

Excerpt from My Journal
November 14, 2011

TODAY BOTH OF US HAD TO RETURN TO WORK. IT WAS VERY difficult to put our fears about cancer to the side and conduct "business as usual." In these circumstances you have to wear a mask of sorts, which covers your real emotions, and do the best you can to interact with people. Hard as it was, there was some comfort in being distracted and focusing on other people. It pulled us outside ourselves. We had one more day to wait until the meeting with the urologist, when many of our questions would be answered.

Both of us did our own exercise regimes, gathered more information on the Internet, and prayed. My husband called some of his friends to share his news. I contacted some of my professional colleagues and requested support, prayer, and resources.

Thoughts About the Topic of Fear

It's important to acknowledge that fear is a typical reaction to a diagnosis of cancer. Cancer is a life-threatening disease, after all. When we hear a cancer diagnosis we are thrown into facing our own mortality or the possible death of our loved one. So it is normal for fears and questions to surface. Acknowledge these fears and questions rather than running from them. If you run from them they only get stronger and more disabling.

Once you contemplate your fears, however, try to put them aside instead of letting them take over your body and/or your mind. Granted, just hearing a diagnosis of prostate cancer is frightening. But fear is often irrational and global in nature. We don't yet know what will happen in the future. **To preserve your sanity and prevent your emotions and body from experiencing a self-induced state of anguish, try saying to yourself:**

I have (or my loved one has) just been given a diagnosis of prostate cancer. I acknowledge that I am frightened, but I will not jump to negative conclusions. I choose to be optimistic and hopeful. We will meet with our doctor and devise a strong treatment plan. In the meantime, I will relax my body and quiet my racing mind by slowing down my breathing, inhaling deeply in my abdomen to a count of four: 1-2-3-4, and exhaling deeply to a count of four: 1-2-3-4. As I breathe and exhale deeply, my mind and body relax. I let go of fear and tension.

If you play your fears over and over in your head you will create a state of anxiety or panic, which will throw you back into the *fight/flight/immobilization* state. If you continue to indulge your fears you will end up depressing your immune system, which is already challenged to maximum capacity in either trying to kill cancer cells (if you're the cancer patient) or helping your loved one.

Anxiety and Panic Attack

Anxiety is a fear-based disorder that occurs when we think about dreadful potential scenarios of the future or become obsessed with guilt about things that have occurred in the past. When you are in a state of anxiety, you lose touch with present time. Your mind goes into the future or the past.

The more your mind imagines horrible things happening in the future or obsesses about guilt from the past, the more frightened and disturbed your body becomes. You will develop the following **symptoms of an anxiety disorder**, which I will explain in layman's terms:

+ Racing mind filled with fear and dread
+ Trouble concentrating
+ Irritability (whether or not you express it)
+ Body feeling agitated
+ Tightness in your head, jaw, neck, shoulders, back
+ Trouble sleeping (falling or staying asleep, or waking up early and not being able to go back to sleep)
+ Pessimistic outlook on life
+ Controlling behavior (aimed at reducing your anxiety)
+ Feeling tired

Staying in a state of anxiety for too long may lead to a panic attack—an intense, terrifying episode of fear that lasts only a short amount of time and can cause the following physical symptoms:

+ Racing heart rate
+ Trouble breathing
+ Discomfort in your stomach
+ Pain in your chest
+ Chills or hot flashes
+ Fear that you are going crazy or losing control of yourself
+ Feeling unsteady

The symptoms of a panic attack are so severe that people often go to the emergency room, thinking they're having a heart attack.

Recommendations for Cancer Patients (and/or Their Loved Ones) Who Are Dealing with Anxiety or Panic Attacks

1. Recognize that anxiety and panic attacks are normal reactions to receiving a diagnosis of cancer (or of having a loved one receive a cancer diagnosis). In this circumstance, cancer is not an imagined fear; it is real and threatening, and it

needs treatment. Your anxiety symptoms should, however, diminish over time.

2. Take power. Do your own research and educate yourself about the severity of the cancer. Use this information to confront your fears—which might tell you that a diagnosis of prostate cancer is a death sentence and that there is no hope. Learn about Gleason scores, clinical stages of prostate cancer, recommended treatment options, and predicted treatment outcomes. *There are many types of treatment available for every stage of prostate cancer.*

3. Plan to meet with your doctor, discuss treatment options, get second opinions, and visit various treatment facilities.

4. Gather a team of people you trust to support you. Fear is strongest when you are isolated.

5. Find some way(s) to release your fears and enjoy the present moment. Among the possibilities: prayer, talking to someone who isn't afraid to hear your fears, journaling, exercising, meditation, yoga, massage therapy, acupuncture, relaxing music, spending time in nature, hanging out with your pet, being of service to someone else in need, gardening, watching uplifting or funny movies, or even doing crossword puzzles.

6. If your symptoms of anxiety or panic attacks persist, find yourself a therapist who can take this journey with you and offer you guidance and support. The therapist might refer you for an evaluation by a psychiatrist, who is a specialist in prescribing anti-anxiety medications. These medications reduce the anxiety or panic to a manageable level, one you can tolerate. The medications are not a sign of weakness on your part but are simply helpful in reducing the anguish of your symptoms, so that you have the energy to fight the cancer. Today's anti-anxiety medications are relatively mild and do not disturb the functioning of your mind or your ability to participate in your normal life.

One more suggestion: If you're like most people, you have some coverage for outpatient mental health care in your medical insurance plan. Use it. Call the number on your insurance card and ask for a referral to a therapist who has experience dealing with cancer. Ask the insurance company about your deductible and co-pay fees per visit.

If you don't have medical and/or mental health insurance, there are therapists and agencies out there that set low, affordable fees. Wellness centers for people who have been diagnosed with cancer are also good sources of support and encouragement, as are hospital cancer support groups. In addition, many hospitals and cancer treatment centers have oncology social workers who can work with you short-term and provide information about community resources. There is no fee for their services. Ask your oncologist for a referral. I found two websites that offer excellent information about cancer counseling: www.cancer.net and www.livestrong.org.

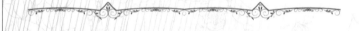

CHAPTER THREE

Learning About Prostate Cancer and Its Treatment Options

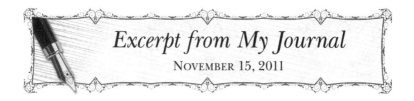

Excerpt from My Journal
NOVEMBER 15, 2011

THIS DAY IS FILLED WITH DREAD AND ANTICIPATION. WE ARE going to meet with the urologist and see the results of the biopsy pathology report. He has set aside forty-five minutes for us to discuss the results and treatment options.

I cannot eat but half my cereal. I cannot drink coffee. I see clients and go to yoga, pick up turkey burgers and salad for dinner—in case we are able to eat this evening.

We try to stay in the moment. I have done research on treatment options, clinical staging, everything I can get my hands on, and have prepared an outline to guide our questions in the doctor's office.

We arrived at the urologist's office at 4:45 p.m. and were ushered into his private study. I want to make a few comments about the interaction. The doctor's face was very gentle, as was his manner. He made eye contact with us as we were seated across from him at his desk. His voice was gentle and compassionate. This human-to-human connection was calming and soothing. He seemed to care about us as human beings and treated us with respect. We both appreciated his manner.

He gave each of us a copy of the four-page pathology report and started to speak. I broke in and told him that I had prepared an outline for questions we wanted to ask, and gave him a copy. He did not seem to mind.

The doctor resumed speaking: "We already knew that your Gleason score was 9 (4+5). What we did not know until now was how many of the core biopsies were involved. On the right lobe of the prostate, five of the six cores were positive for cancer; 60%. The diagnosis on the right lobe is: prostatic adenocarcinoma, poorly differentiated. Predicted Gleason score 4+5=9 of 10. Focal intraprostatic perineural invasion noted into the left lobe. Focal high-grade PIN also present. No extracapsular soft tissue is identified for determination of extracapsular invasion.

"On the left lobe of the prostate, one of the six cores was positive for cancer; 2%. The diagnosis is: microfocal prostatic adeno-carcinoma, poorly differentiated. Predicted Gleason score 4+4=8 of 10."

We did not fully understand this explanation at the time, and the doctor had a lot more to talk about, so when we got home I studied the second page of the pathology report, which explains the Gleason score:

> *For prostate cancer, the grade is the single most powerful prognostic indicator, or in other words, the most impor-tant piece of information used to predict how likely a given cancer is to spread. The grading system most widely used in prostate cancer is the "Gleason grade" or "Gleason score," named after its inventor, Dr. Donald Gleason.*
>
> *Prostate cancers grow in certain patterns. There are five Gleason patterns, designated 1-5. Pattern 1 shows a uni-formity of growth which is quite similar in appearance to normal prostate gland structures, but is rarely ever seen. Pro-ceeding down through patterns 2-5, the cancer structures show progressively more irregular shapes, and it is these pro-gressive irregularities that were originally demonstrated by Dr. Gleason to correlate with cancer aggressiveness, with pattern 5 being the most aggressive.*
>
> *The Gleason score is arrived at by the pathologist adding the two most common Gleason patterns present in a given cancer, always indicating the most prevalent, or primary*

pattern first. For example, a cancer which is mostly pattern 3 and has lesser areas of pattern 4 would be given a Gleason score "3+4=7." A cancer having only a pattern 3 would be assigned a Gleason score "3+3=6."

Importantly, the Gleason score correlates in a predictive fashion with other significant pathologic and clinical features. Specifically, the higher the Gleason score, the higher are the risks of extraprostatic extension, seminal vesicle invasion, lymph node metastasis, and the probability of disease recurrence after treatment.

The term "differentiation" can be used almost interchangeably with Gleason score, where "well differentiated" means Gleason score 2-4, "moderately differentiated" means Gleason scores 5 or 6, and "poorly differentiated" includes Gleason scores 8-10.

Meanwhile, back in the doctor's office, my husband and I were overwhelmed with the information we were hearing. We sat there with wide eyes, barely breathing. The news was worse than we expected. Finally my husband was able to whisper, "What is the treatment for this kind of cancer? My cousin had a Gleason score of 6 and only had to have radiation therapy. That's what I would like to do."

The doctor gently responded:

"I don't recommend that you have radiation therapy now. That is something we might think about later. Because your Gleason score is 9 and your cancer is so aggressive,

the best hope for cure is for you to have surgery. There are two types of surgery you could have:

1. Traditional, open radical prostatectomy, where I would do one long incision and remove your prostate, pelvic lymph nodes, and seminal vesicles. You would be hospitalized for seven to ten days, and there is the risk of blood loss, 5 percent risk of incontinence, 60 to 70 percent risk of erectile dysfunction.

2. The newer robotic-assisted radical prostatectomy, which would make a number of small incisions to allow the robot and the surgeon to remove the prostate, pelvic lymph nodes, and seminal vesicles. You would be hospitalized for two to three days, and there would be less risk of blood loss, same risk of infection, incontinence, and erectile dysfunction."

This information was frightening too. Erectile dysfunction and incontinence were two of my husband's greatest fears.

The doctor went on to say: "Before we make any plan I would like to order some tests—a bone scan and a CT scan of the abdomen and pelvis, with contrast—to determine if the cancer has spread outside the prostate."

By this point we had been in the office close to an hour, and we were both exhausted. The doctor asked his office manager to arrange the tests, and she was able to schedule us for two days from now. We shook everyone's hand and walked out of the office. Both of us could barely walk the long way to the car.

When we talked in the car on the ride home, I voiced my opinion about the treatment choices:

> *"Because of the high Gleason score and the aggressiveness of this type of cancer, I agree with the doctor that you should have surgery. I think it is important to get this cancer out of your body as soon as possible. You don't want to give it a chance to grow outside the prostate capsule. Radiation therapy is done over a course of eight to nine weeks, which would give the cancer a chance to spread."*

My husband responded:

> *"I don't want to have surgery, but if I have to have it I would choose the robotic-assisted radical prostatectomy. There is less blood loss, less time spent in the hospital, less chance of infection. But I don't like hearing about the high potential for incontinence and erectile dysfunction. I would still rather have radiation."*

When we got home we did more talking, and both of us were encouraged that there were many different treatment options, now and in the future. The doctor said he recommended surgery for now, but in the future we also had the options of radiation and hormone therapy. The doctor stated that many men with this high-risk prostate cancer go on to live long lives. With this encouragement and hope, we were able to eat our turkey burgers and went to bed early.

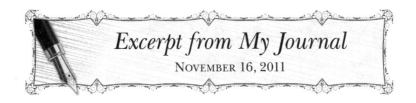

Excerpt from My Journal
November 16, 2011

*I WAKE UP AT 3:30 A.M. AND THE SPIRIT IS GIVING ME A VISU-
alization to share with my husband:*

> *"The walls of the prostate are thick, strong, flexible, made
> of titanium. They are able to contain the hyper, confused,
> undifferentiated cancer cells. There are also healthy white
> cells inside the prostate, and we are going to make them
> stronger with good nutrition, love, the power of God, and
> therapy. We are going to starve the cancer by going on a
> low-fat, high-natural-grain, fruit-and-vegetable diet. We
> are going to change the molecular structure of all the cells.
> We can do it.*
>
> *Our team of helpers is outside the prostate, ready to install
> a powerful protective lining around it and a flexible,
> stainless steel border all around the perimeter—which
> will prevent the cancer from breaching the prostate cap-
> sule. Our team is composed of our dog Brutie, our
> children and grandchildren, our brothers, our friends,
> God, Jesus, the Spirit, the doctors, the treatment, Silent
> Unity, and my colleagues.*
>
> *God is with us. Spirit is talking to us and guiding us
> each step of the way. We will win the fight against*

prostate cancer and we will share our experience with others. We and our marriage will continue. Our lives will continue. There is no need to be afraid. We are safe and we are strong."

When I wake up with a bad case of diarrhea, I realize that I must put the cancer to the side today and take care of myself. Fortunately my noon client cancelled and I had most of the day to myself. I took a hot bath, read a bit, and took a nap with Brutie, our puppy. I needed to be quiet; to allow my body to rest and release the built-up tension.

I recorded this dream when I woke up:

> "Inside the house I was installing Christmas-like lights throughout to brighten the darkness. The man who lived there was rather small and needed assistance from other men to walk. We brought him into the house, and he was delighted and encouraged to see the lights."

In analyzing this dream, I think the small man represented both my animus (my masculine side in Jungian psychology terms)—who was holding so much stress and fear and had to handle so many cancer-related tasks; and my husband, whose size was temporarily diminished by the fear and threat of cancer, and who needed the support of other men who have been treated for prostate cancer, along with his male family members and friends who love him. The lights that I was installing in the house represented the power of God and medicine and our own powerful spirits to conquer the cancer, give us hope, and make us feel safe in the darkness that was encroaching upon us.

Dealing with cancer is stressful and fatiguing. Being the wife of the husband recently diagnosed with prostate cancer is a very sharp learning curve. I don't know anything about the prostate, the seminal vesicles. Thank goodness I have prior experience as an oncology social worker, which gives me at least some understanding of the medical system. Never did I imagine I would have a husband who would develop cancer. That is the part I was NOT prepared for: being a family member caring for a cancer patient.

Because I love my husband with all my heart, I am trying to remove the stress from his body and usher him through the medical maze. At home I want him to feel safe, loved, and cherished. I encourage him to talk about anything and everything, and I share my thoughts and feelings as well.

It is comforting to sleep together. I am soothed by cuddling against his body, and the proximity allows me to touch him and pray for him throughout the night. Tomorrow we are going for two tests, the CT scan and the bone scan. We need to find out if the prostate cancer has penetrated its capsule and is detectable in any other part of the body. I pray with all my heart that it has not; that it is safely contained in the prostate. Obviously we want to begin treatment as soon as possible. This aggressive form of cancer should be removed as soon as possible!

Before I go to sleep I write a prayer in my journal:

Dearest Lord,

As I have told You, we are both in the palm of Your Hand. We are small, we are scared, we are in need of a miracle. Please continue to guide and comfort us. I pray the cancer has not spread; that the prostate capsule is strong and resistant to penetration. We are already making dietary changes. Please assist us with access to the doctors and scheduling for treatment as soon as possible. We give You thanks for being part of our family and praise You for Your Love. We are Your kids.

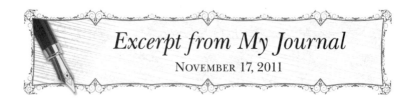

Excerpt from My Journal
November 17, 2011

Today we spent the day at St. John's Hospital. I was happy to be there, in familiar surroundings from my past. I had no fear of the hospital, the staff, the procedures, and was glad to be at my husband's side, assisting with the coordination of tasks. I know that my presence and confidence enabled him to relax and lean on me.

I had never seen the preparation for a bone scan. One hour before the test, my husband was injected with radioactive dye and had to drink a quart of a barium mixture, which tasted awful. My husband was smart to drink it slowly so that he did not gag or throw up. After that he was taken into another department for his CT scan.

While I waited for him I went to the front desk and told the clerk we wanted to get copies of the bone scan and CT scan for our own records. The clerk told me my husband would have to sign a release of information and that she would prepare the scans and their reports on a CD, which we could pick up the following day.

The doctor had also recommended that we sign a release to have the Pathology Department find, prepare, and release my husband's biopsy slides, which we would need if we went for any second-opinion consultations. I mentioned this to the clerk, and she directed me to go down on the elevator to the Pathology Department. I followed her directions and arrived at the Pathology Department, where they allowed me to place the order on the condition that my husband sign the release once the slides were ready to pick up.

Back on the main floor I phoned the urologist and asked more questions about the robotic-assisted radical prostatectomy. He recommended that we go to City of Hope (a world-famous cancer treatment center) and transferred me to his office manager, who gave me the phone number of the surgeon's appointment coordinator for new patients. When my husband completed his tests, we called City of Hope and were fortunate to schedule a consultative appointment with the surgeon on the following Wednesday. In the meantime I had to fax the office manager the pathology report and promise we would arrive with the pathology slides, paper reports, and CD of the scans.

This day at the hospital gave me a sense of immense satisfaction. I was "back in the saddle," working as an oncology social worker—making phone calls, scheduling appointments, collecting reports. I was happy that I could be of assistance to my husband and facilitate a speedy approach to treatment.

My husband and I actually had a good day of working together. We laughed as we rode the elevator from floor to floor and kissed outside in the sun, under the beautiful green trees on the St. John's terrace. I reminded him that we were "One Person, Four Feet."

We went to the deli, our new home, and were both starving from not eating all day. We ate ravenously and were delighted our bodies would allow us to enjoy and tolerate the food.

Last night I began reading Anticancer: A New Way of Life, *by David Servan-Schreiber, M.D., Ph.D. The book had been recommended to me by a friend and colleague who is a naturopathic doctor in Portland, Oregon—Dr. Shani Fox—who specializes in the treatment of cancer. On her advice I ordered the book on Amazon and watched a brief YouTube video of Dr. Servan-Schreiber on his Amazon page. Dr. Servan-Schreiber is himself a fifteen-year survivor of brain cancer, with one relapse. I am eager to read the latest research and theories on treating cancer with a holistic approach. I am sure there has been a lot of progress since I was an oncology social worker in the 1970s.*

The Spirit was with us throughout the day. All the scheduling of appointments and getting copies of the scans, reports, and pathology slides fell into place like clockwork. Truly we are blessed, and God is with us. To top things off, this was the affirmation in Daily Word today:

> *"The Spirit of God goes before me, making safe and successful my way."*

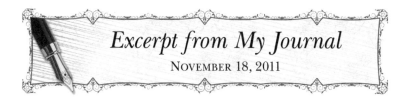

Excerpt from My Journal
NOVEMBER 18, 2011

YESTERDAY, WHILE WAITING IN THE HOSPITAL, I FINALLY HAD the courage to read the whole pathology report and look at the pictures of the cancer cells. It was very frightening to see them—these Gleason 9 cancer cells. They are dark and swirling with activity, menacing and very dangerous. The fact that they are "undifferentiated" makes them even more dangerous. They do not grow in circle shapes, like the normal cells. These cells are misshaped, dark in color, and independent in nature—which means it is easier for them to break out of the prostate and escape to other parts of the body.

I began to wonder about the power of prayer to change the shape and characteristics of the cancer cells. Later that day the Spirit gave me an extension for my husband's visualization imagery:

"Through the power of God working in our lives and the power of prayer, we are able to cast out the malicious intent in the cancer cells.

God's love and healing power are manifesting as Light that is entering the prostate capsule. The Light is surrounding each and every undifferentiated cancer cell and releasing the anger and danger they possess. They become a lighter color. They become calmer and stationary. Slowly, the Light gathers them into larger and larger circles so that their structure resembles the shape of normal cells. They lose their potency and danger.

Meanwhile, the healthy cells become stronger and more robust through the power of God, prayer, lack of fear, and the changes we will make in our diet. The normal cells begin to surround the newly formed cancer clusters. They forgive the cancer cells for their invasion and go about doing what they were designed to do. They eat the cancer cells and send their waste out of the body, through the organs of elimination. We have already deprived the cancer cells of the foods and conditions they thrive on by eating anti-cancer foods, vitamins, and supplements."

You can imagine my amazement later in the day when I read the following quote in the Anticancer *book, on page 36:*

"Natural killer (NK) cells are very special agents of the immune system. Like all white blood cells, they patrol the organism continually in search of bacteria, viruses, or

new cancer cells. But while other cells of the immune system need previous exposure to disease agents in order to recognize and combat them, NK cells don't need prior introduction to an antigen in order to mobilize. As soon as they detect an enemy, they gather around the intruders, seeking membrane-to-membrane contact. Once they make contact, NK cells aim their internal equipment at their target, like a tank turret. This equipment carries vesicles filled with poisons.

On contact with the cancer cell's surface, the vesicles are released and the chemical weapons of the NK cells—perforin and granzymes—penetrate the membrane. The molecules of perforin take the shape of tiny circles, or microrings. They are assembled in the shape of a tube, forming a passage for the granzymes through the cancer cell's membrane. At the core of the cancer cell, the granzymes then activate the mechanisms of programmed self-destruction. It's as if they give the cancer cell an order to commit suicide, an order it has no choice but to obey. In response to this message, its nucleus crumbles, leading to the cancer cell's collapse. The deflated remains of the cell are then ready to be digested by microphages, which are the garbage collectors of the immune system and are always found in the wake of NK cells."

Isn't God amazing? In the quiet of my bedroom He sent the Spirit, who gave me the expanded visualization for my husband—which correlates directly with the most current cancer research! This may seem amazing but, in truth, God has assisted me in this way throughout my life and in my work with clients.

I found another helpful quote in the Anticancer *book, on page 40:*

> "...*Cancer cells will flourish only within an individual whose immune defenses have been weakened. It may be primarily the lack of healthy defenses that allows otherwise dormant cancer cells to become aggressive tumors. ... Studies on the activity of immune cells (including NK cells and white blood cells targeted against cancer) show that they are at their best when our diets are healthy, our environment is 'clean,' and our physical activity involves the entire body (not just our brains and our hands). Immune cells are also sensitive to our emotions. They react positively to emotional states characterized by a sense of well-being and a feeling that we are connected to those around us."*

My husband told me today:

> "*Somehow I never thought I would die. It's something that only happens to other people. The thought that I have cancer is humbling. I am hoping I can qualify for proton therapy at Loma Linda Hospital. I would like not to have surgery. I could live with lack of sexual functioning, but I am afraid to be left with incontinence."*

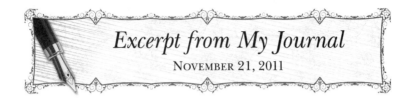

Excerpt from My Journal
NOVEMBER 21, 2011

THANK YOU, HEAVENLY FATHER. WE MET WITH OUR UROLOGIST today, and the CT scan and the bone scan were NEGATIVE! No signs of cancer outside the prostate! The whole-body bone imaging study said: "No apparent metastatic disease to the skeleton." The CT of the abdomen and pelvis with contrast concluded: "No evidence of invasion of bladder or rectum. No evidence of pelvic lymphadenopathy."

We were both so overjoyed with the excellent news. My husband said: "I am ready to move ahead with the robotic-assisted prostatectomy at City of Hope. My urologist highly recommended the surgeon there, and I will put my trust in him. My urologist will follow me after the surgery and coordinate with the surgeon."

Through this statement, I observed in my husband a reaction that I will now call his "modus operandi." When he is first presented with an option he does not like, his first response is to say "no." What I am beginning to understand now is that he does not mean "no, forever." He is really saying "no, not right now." Because of the way his mind works, he is the kind of guy who needs more information and more time to make the right decision. He wants someone to convince him with facts. Once he receives the facts he will take his time to digest the information, and if the facts are compelling enough he will change his mind. That's a pretty neat quality!

We are both so relieved. We could not stop expressing, "Praise God! Praise God!" This morning each of us had diarrhea prior to our meeting with the doctor.

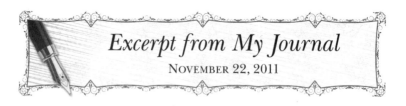

Excerpt from My Journal
NOVEMBER 22, 2011

MORE EXCELLENT NEWS: MY ROUTINE, EVERY-FIVE-YEAR colonoscopy today was excellent—no cancer or polyps observed. I happily celebrated with leftover Indian food and am resting in bed with Brutie. So far the stress from the cancer is not causing any problems in my own body.

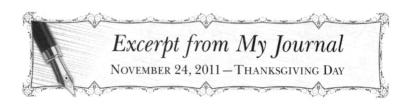

Excerpt from My Journal
NOVEMBER 24, 2011 — THANKSGIVING DAY

DEAREST LORD,

Today I am quietly and not so quietly freaking out. We went to see the surgeon at City of Hope yesterday and I have mixed feelings about our visit.

The good news is that the surgeon agreed the robotic-assisted radical prostatectomy is the best course of action to take. My husband is scheduled for his pre-op on Monday at 9:40 a.m. and his surgery on Tuesday. This is really blessed intervention, as the surgeon's earliest available surgery opening had been December 20 but a last-minute cancellation gave us the spot on November 29.

We thank You for that and for another blessed break: getting the pre-op appointment on November 28. Again there were no openings, but I implored the scheduling nurse to get my husband in. I was bold enough to grab the Sacred Heart of Jesus medal around my neck, show it to her, and say: "Jesus wants him to get an appointment on November 28. Without it he cannot have his surgery on November 29, and he has a very aggressive case of prostate cancer. He cannot wait."

I knew I was taking a chance to be that assertive, but I was willing to do anything necessary to help my husband. It was not the time to be timid. His life depended on the surgery, as soon as possible!

We gave the scheduling nurse our cell phone number, and as we were driving home in the car she phoned us and said: "I am able to give you the pre-op appointment on November 28. I called the first man on the list, who was scheduled for surgery at a later date than your husband, and he said he was happy to give you his appointment. I have rescheduled his pre-op appointment for a later date."

All of this is very good news. The immediate challenge we are facing is that my husband began coming down with a very bad cold yesterday, and we have only four days to get him well enough to pass his pre-op exam. This will be especially difficult because it was the surgeon's opinion and order that he should not take Advil, Aleve, aspirin, or any vitamin supplements.

Please help us. We are desperate to get this cancer out as soon as possible. We can only rely on You.

What was unsettling about our talk with the surgeon was that he seemed to stress the gravity of the Gleason 9 score: "This is a very high-risk cancer. There is a great possibility that it has metastasized elsewhere in the body. We won't really know until we operate and I can see what the prostate looks like, and biopsy the pelvic lymph nodes and seminal vesicles."

This is all scary information, my Lord, and yesterday and this morning I was really feeling overwhelmed: "What is going to happen to us and our life? What will the surgical biopsies reveal? What are we going to do?"

Another thing we did not like was that the surgeon was pushing my husband to join one of his three clinical trials. City of Hope is a teaching and research center, and we could understand the surgeon's interest in our participation. We appreciated the idea of his trials but wished he had spent less time discussing them and more time focusing on us and our needs, concerns, and questions. We declined the trials, as one of them might have delayed surgery by six weeks while my hus-

band underwent a round of chemotherapy (unless he was in the control group that would receive only a placebo), and another one required that he return for a series of blood draws after the surgery—which was inconvenient because of the two-hour-round-trip commute.

I am also feeling frustrated by my husband's resistance to giving up red meat and to exercising a half-hour per day—suggestions that were made in a second book I am reading, entitled Life Over Cancer, by Keith I. Block of the Block Center for Integrative Cancer Treatment. "How could he not do this if it will increase his chances of beating cancer?" I found myself getting angry at him. "I do not want a life without him...." Then I realized it is his life, and I cannot police or control it. He must be in charge of his own life. I can only make suggestions, offer advice, put the literature before him, pray for and with him, love him, encourage him, model holistic behavior to him, and let go.

Letting go is so difficult, Lord. We need You every moment to show us the way and lead our every step. **I DO NOT WANT TO LOSE MY HUSBAND!** Please, please help us.

Thank You for guiding me to Psalm 40,1-3:

> "I waited patiently for God to help me; then He listened and heard my cry. He lifted me out of the pit of despair, out from the bog and the mire, and set my feet on a hard, firm path and steadied me as I walked along. He has given me a new song to sing, of praises to our God. Now

many will hear of the glorious things He did for me, and stand in awe before the Lord, and put their trust in Him."

Fixing the Thanksgiving meal this year was a real challenge. I didn't have much energy, my head was in a blur, and I wanted to make a healthier meal with foods that supported the anti-cancer diet recommendations I had been reading about. I chose to eliminate certain "traditional" items from the menu: white mashed potatoes, gravy, stuffing, commercial pies, white-flour biscuits. Instead I substituted baked yams, Caesar salad, brown rice, whole-wheat biscuits, and a recipe for sautéed kale with lemon and raw walnuts, which my daughter obtained from the Prostate Cancer Foundation. She baked a pumpkin pie from a recipe she found on the same website. My husband was okay with most of the changes, but he insisted on his traditional jellied cranberry sauce. We served sparkling cider instead of wine.

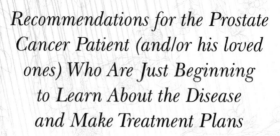

Recommendations for the Prostate Cancer Patient (and/or his loved ones) Who Are Just Beginning to Learn About the Disease and Make Treatment Plans

1. As you begin to navigate the medical system, **buy a large folder with pockets** that will hold all of the reports, test results, and meeting notes from your visits with each doctor. It is very important for you to have your own files so that you can study them at your leisure. My husband and I, in fact, kept our own separate files.

   When you're going for a second- or third-opinion consultation, make copies of your reports to give to the new doctor. It often takes too much time for one doctor or one institution to send copies of reports to another doctor.

   Ask your doctors (urologist, surgeon, radiation oncologist, medical oncologist) for copies of their transcribed notes from each visit. Doctors and hospitals are required to oblige your request for documents but often don't *offer* to give you copies.

   You will also want to keep copies of articles you obtain from the Internet. I was surprised when some doctors, who were not up to speed with the current research findings, asked for copies of my articles.

2. **"The squeaky wheel gets oiled."** This mentality is *critical* for you to remember—and put into practice. You must be your own advocate, and you must learn to be assertive. When you're dealing with cancer you don't have time to be timid, laid back, or hopeful that someone else is going to take care of you.

You must be willing to make phone calls to schedule appointments, coordinate one doctor with another, keep things rolling forward. In large hospital systems it's easy to be overlooked or placed at the end of a waiting list. I'm not suggesting that you be obnoxious or rude to anyone; but you need to assertively keep after the staff until you accomplish your objective. This is your life, your body, your cancer (or your loved one's, as the case may be).

Within a ten-day period from the point of diagnosis, we were able to gather the following information about my husband's cancer. Because he had a very aggressive form of prostate cancer, it was imperative to obtain this information within the shortest amount of time possible—so that we could expedite the treatment decision:

MY HUSBAND'S PROSTATE CANCER PROFILE

MOST RECENT PSA: 6

RESULTS OF BIOPSY PATHOLOGY REPORT

GLEASON SCORE

8-10: *called "poorly differentiated or high-grade"*
Right lobe: *4+5=9 of 10*
Left lobe: *4+4=8 of 10*

PERCENTAGE OF CORE BIOPSIES POSITIVE FOR CANCER

Right lobe: *Estimated 60% of biopsy tissue involved*
(5 positive of 6 cores)

Left lobe: *Estimated 2% of biopsy tissue involved*
(1 positive of 6 cores)

TYPE OF CANCER

Right lobe: *Prostatic adenocarcinoma, poorly differentiated*
Focal intraprostatic perineural invasion into left lobe

Left lobe: *Microfocal prostatic adenocarcinoma,*
poorly differentiated

DIAGNOSTIC TESTS RESULTS

1. *CT SCAN OF PELVIS: negative for bladder and rectum*
   No pelvic lymphadenopathy
2. *BONE SCAN: negative*

3. **Don't be afraid to tell the doctor that you don't understand what he is saying.** Ask questions and seek further clarification. There are no dumb questions. You are not a medical professional and are not expected to understand medical terminology or procedures. It's a good idea to write down questions before each doctor visit. If you forget to bring something up, cover it on your next visit.

4. **Reserve the right to make your own decisions about treatment.** Do not automatically proceed with the doctor's recommendations. Again, it is your body, your risk from side effects, your point of view (or your loved one's, as the case may be). Listen to the doctor's recommendations and discuss the options. It might be helpful to take a tape recorder to each visit and ask the doctor if you can record the conversation, so that you can analyze it once you get home. Often there is just too much information to grasp in the doctor's office.

It's important that you do your own research and visit the various medical centers to find out where you're most comfortable and confident. In *Anticancer*, Dr. David Servan-Schreiber notes that when he was choosing the doctor to treat his brain cancer, he chose one who was the most compassionate and approachable over someone who might have been a better technician.

5. **Give yourself emotional and psychological support.** Neither of the first two doctors we visited suggested that we see a therapist to be evaluated for anxiety and depression or to receive emotional and psychological support in our fight against cancer. I was shocked! This oversight was the norm in the 1970s, but I was alarmed to see that nothing was different in 2011.

When I asked if City of Hope had oncology social workers or used alternative therapy approaches, I was told that the facility only provides a dietician for those patients who are receiving radiation therapy, and that it only offers yoga and art therapy once a week. No oncology social workers were mentioned.

I am very serious when I tell you that you will need emotional and psychological support. Even though I'm a trained professional in the field of social work and psychotherapy and can offer a lot of assistance to my husband, I'm humble and experienced enough to realize that I, too, needed help in this journey. Living with cancer is extremely challenging and overwhelming. I believe that, as the loved one of a cancer patient, if you don't reach out for support you will be at high risk for developing cancer or some other illness. As a patient, meantime, I believe that if you don't receive support, your immune system will be depressed and your chances of beating the cancer will drop.

6. **Tap into the power of prayer.** I have learned over the course of my lifetime that God is available to guide our steps, give us counsel, and create blessings for us. We only have to ask. I'm not suggesting that you have to belong to a particular religion. I believe that God presents Himself in different forms to people around the world. You don't have to attend a church in order to pray. You can do it in the privacy of your own home and your own heart, in your own way.

In my personal experience God always comes through. He magnifies my own personal power and abilities, lifting me up when I am down or lost or discouraged. In the treatment of cancer He creates opportunities for scheduling appointments when none exist; directs us to the right treatment providers; and helps our bodies, minds, emotions, and spirits to heal. If you've never prayed or you don't believe in God, you have nothing to lose. Give it a chance, step back, and see what happens.

7. **Visualizations and positive affirmations are powerful techniques in the fight against cancer.** Research has proven that what we think in our minds has a corresponding effect on our bodies and emotions. If you expect a negative outcome, it will likely materialize; it's called the *self-fulfilling prophecy.* Similarly, if you expect a positive outcome *it* will likely materialize.

Earlier in this chapter I shared some of the visualizations that the Spirit gave us during the first part of our cancer journey. By their nature, visualizations and affirmations are positive thoughts that produce positive reactions within the systems of the body—enhancing healing and repair. Visualizations and affirmations lower our heart rate and blood pressure and make the immune system more effective. They give us a sense of power, hope, and calm. They can be especially helpful when we're trying to go to sleep, when we're struggling to stay asleep, or when we're experiencing anxiety or panic attacks. They are produced by the mind, but their effects ripple through every part of our body, our conscious and our unconscious. Visualizations can be fun and creative, and they sure beat the alternative of a panic attack!

8. **Work together as a team.** Whether you're the cancer patient or the patient's loved one, remember that you are a team. Each of you will have your own strengths to contribute. Respect your individual differences and capitalize on your unique gifts. Listen to one another with patience, and don't be afraid to express your real emotions or fears to each other.

If you're the loved one of a prostate cancer patient, you must defer to him. Offer your suggestions and recommendations, but know when to back off and let go. Ultimately the patient must make the final treatment choices. It's his body and his life. Continue to love and support him, even if you disagree. Concentrate on keeping yourself healthy and calm.

9. **Don't expect that medical treatment alone will cure the cancer.** As soon as possible after diagnosis, **take your personal power and look at ways you can enhance health and healing through exercise, diet, and mindfulness practices.**

Exercise. Do some form of cardio exercise for at least a half-hour a day. Exercise will decrease your stress and tension, release endorphins ("feel good" hormones), and make you feel stronger and more confident.

A beginner-level yoga class will teach you deep abdominal breathing, ground you in your body, quiet your anxiety, build your strength, and gently stretch your tight muscles and spine. These activities will, in turn, give flexibility to your thinking and reacting. If you're not interested in yoga try Tai Chi, weight training, swimming, using an elliptical machine or treadmill, cycling—activities that won't put too much stress on the spine, abdomen, and pelvis.

If you're the prostate cancer patient, the level of exercise you choose depends on what type of treatment you're receiving as well as your doctor's approval. **If you have a low Gleason score** and are being treated only with "active surveillance," you can engage in more strenuous exercise like martial arts or heavier weight training or longer-distance aerobic exercises. **If you're recovering from surgery**, your body needs at least six weeks to heal. So your exercise should be less strenuous, and any weightlifting you do should be light. **If you are undergoing radiation treatment for eight to nine weeks**, your body might be sore and you may be challenged by fatigue. So again, your exercise should not be strenuous. **If you are undergoing long-term**

androgen deprivation therapy, your doctor should evaluate your bone density/brittleness, cardiac health, and diabetes, if you have it. Generally, some form of weight-bearing exercise will make the most sense for you; it will make your bones stronger, keep your weight down, and reduce the size of your abdomen.

Diet. The books *Life Over Cancer* and *Anticancer* both describe scientific evidence showing that diet affects the growth of cancer cells. Reading these books, you will see that **certain foods promote cancer growth and increase inflammation throughout the body**: sugar, fat, refined white flour and pasta, white rice, animal protein (especially red meat), fried foods, dairy products.

By the same token, **certain foods retard cancer growth and enhance the functioning of your immune system**: whole grains (whole-wheat bread and pasta, brown rice, oats, barley, millet, quinoa, buckwheat), soy products, fatty fish rich in omega-3, vegetables with a variety of colors, leafy greens, cruciferous vegetables (Brussels sprouts, broccoli, cauliflower, kale, onions, garlic), mushrooms, legumes, yams, a multitude of fruits (especially berries of all kinds, kiwi, apples, melons, apples, and avocados), olive oil, flaxseed oil, canola oil, omega-3 butter, cod liver oil, seaweed, nuts and seeds (like walnuts, hazelnuts, pecans, and almonds), green tea, and herbs and spices (turmeric, curry, mint, thyme, marjoram, oregano, basil and rosemary, parsley and celery, leeks, shallots, chives, cinnamon, and ginger). Some research also suggests moderate use (one glass per day) of red wine—which contains the antioxidant resveratrol—and dark chocolate (more than 70 percent cocoa). You can also focus on using natural sweeteners (agave, Stevia, rice syrup) instead of sugar, honey, and artificial sweeteners.

For a complete list of anti-cancer foods and an explanation of how they work, I suggest that you simply go ahead and buy *Life Over Cancer* and *Anticancer*. When you read these books you'll see, for example, that the latest research indicates my husband's urologist was mistaken in restricting all chocolate and spicy foods.

The key here is to make the dietary transition gradually. As my husband put it: "You have to cut me some slack. I am a foodie, and this is hard for me. I'm willing to make some changes, but I have to do it in my own time. Don't worry if I eat or drink some of the bad things. You may lose some of the food battles in order to win the war. It's a long-term thing."

Mindfulness practices. Try to spend some time each day being quiet with yourself and turning inward. In the silence you'll begin to recognize the voice of your spirit—that part of you which connects to Higher Power. Some people call it *intuition*. It's the gentle voice that gives you guidance, comfort, encouragement, and strength.

I begin my spiritual time in the morning. I take my dog, Brutie, for a one-hour walk and connect with nature. Brutie is the best antidepressant: we run, we play, we laugh together, we kiss. I see the birds, the trees, the flowers, the sky, my neighbors, other dogs. I feel the sun and wind on my face and body. My focus is outside my head, beyond my problems. I stay in the moment. This is a form of *mindfulness*.

When we return to the house I fix Brutie's breakfast and then eat mine outside—in my front garden. I read the day's passage in *Daily Word* and have my prayer time. I connect with my spirit. This ritual ensures that I have some control and comfort in my daily life, despite what is going on with the cancer.

Meditation is another valuable tool for self-care. According to Kelly McGonigal, Ph.D., author of

The Willpower Instinct, a UCLA research team led by Eileen Luders has documented that **people who meditate regularly experience improvements in the structure and functioning of their brains**. Meditation increases the density of the hippocampus (which improves memory and helps reduce and regulate stress). The brain stem (which controls the autonomic nervous system and the fight/flight response) calms down during meditation. Meditation also increases the density of the gray and white matter in the prefrontal cortex (an area of the brain that handles decision making, self-awareness, impulse control, and the regulation of distractions). Research shows, too, that the particular type of meditation you do (Buddhist, yoga, or secular) isn't important; good results emerge from many different approaches to the practice. And people who are new to meditation achieve positive results within a short period of time.

I leave you with this thought: **stress = cortisol release = inflammation = depressed immune system = cancer cell growth.**

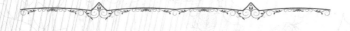

CHAPTER FOUR

Robotic-Assisted Radical Prostatectomy

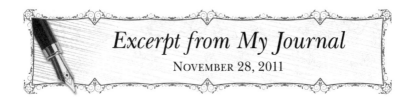

Excerpt from My Journal

NOVEMBER 28, 2011

TODAY WE MADE THE EIGHTY-MILE-ROUND-TRIP DRIVE TO CITY of Hope for my husband's pre-op evaluation. Thank God the cold he had been battling cycled from his nose to his throat to his chest in four days, and his coughing subsided. This was a little miracle as historically this type of cold can last for three weeks to a month.

At the hospital, we were directed from one department to another for X-ray, EKG, lab work, and a meeting with the anesthesiologist. Finally we met with the surgeon's nurse practitioner, who said my husband had been cleared for surgery the following day. She gave us a preview of what to expect:

+ *No food or drink after midnight.*

+ *Take one shower tonight and one in the morning.*

+ *Arrive at the hospital by 9:30 a.m. Your surgery is scheduled for 11:00 a.m.*

+ *The surgery will be done by the surgeon and the 2005 da Vinci robot. The surgeon sits at a console and manipulates the arms of the robot, whose "hands" enter the body through the incision sites, along with a camera. The surgical team assists the operation.*

+ *When you arrive you will be admitted to the pre-surgery area, and you will be there for approximately one and a half hours.*

+ *The surgeon will talk to you briefly, then you will be wheeled into surgery. You will be placed on a reclining table, with your head down, in a supine position. The surgery will take approximately three and a half hours. The surgeon will make six small incisions in the abdominal area and a larger one under the belly button to remove the prostate, lymph nodes, and seminal vesicles. The surgeon will use surgical glue to close the incisions and insert a Foley catheter into the penis. You will have a puffy face, from the inclined position of your head, and pain from your shoulders to your diaphragm. You will be on antibiotics and pain medication.*

+ *After the surgery you will be monitored in the recovery room for two hours to make sure there are no complica-*

tions. When you are cleared you will be moved to your private room, located in a wing devoted to men with prostate cancer, and you will stay there overnight. You will be encouraged to walk as soon as possible. Walking will aid the recovery process.

+ *If there are no complications you will be discharged home the next day. The nurse will instruct your wife on how to take care of the Foley catheter, which you must wear for one week. You will also have a drain tube to remove fluids from the abdominal area.*

+ *You are to call the triage nurse here if you have any problems with your catheter, experience pain that does not go away with Percocet or Vicodin, have a fever over 100, or experience nausea or vomiting. Take Colace and Metamucil as stool softeners and Extra Strength Tylenol as needed. You will be on the antibiotic Levaquin.*

+ *You will return to see the surgeon in one week, and he will inspect your incisions and determine if the catheter can be removed.*

When we finally returned to our house I was tense, frightened, and tired. As I thought about the strain I was feeling, the ten-to eleven-hour day coming up, and the fear of what the surgeon might find once opening my husband up, I felt overwhelmed. My husband had his own emotions going on and wanted to talk to alleviate his anxiety. I told him I did not have the energy to talk and wanted to get to bed quickly. I told him I was *exhausted, feeling the strain, and did not want to be grouchy with him. He snapped, "You switch from friendly and accessible to silent. I don't like it. **I'm** the patient!" I knew he felt hurt, but there was nothing more I could do. "He'll just have to handle his own emotions and prepare for the surgery," I thought. "I **must** get some sleep."*

I thought to myself:

> *"He is the patient, but I feel like the patient too. My world has been turned upside down too. We are One Person, Four Legs. He will be operated on, but I have to drive us safely, get us there on time, shepherd him while we wait, pray for him those three to four hours, telephone our family and prayer partners, pray until we hear from the doctor, phone our people again, encourage and care for him in his room, make the long drive home in the dark, comfort our puppy who has been waiting all day alone, get ready to bring him home the next day, and take care of his medical, emotional, mental, and spiritual needs. I must get some rest and pray myself to sleep or I won't be able to cope."*

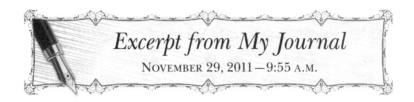

Excerpt from My Journal

NOVEMBER 29, 2011—9:55 A.M.

DEAREST LORD,

Here we are at the pre-surgery station. We are very thankful to be here so quickly and to be so well taken care of. We were remarking that only two and a half weeks ago we received the fateful phone call: "Gleason score 9." So much has happened so quickly—all the parts falling into place. Thank You for taking such good care of us. Thank You for family who are supporting us with their love and prayers. Thank You for so many "state of grace" days during this period.

Please let my husband be without fear, experience no infection, and retain as much sexual and bladder function as is safely possible. Bless the surgeon and the staff throughout the long procedure.

Help us to "stay in the moment" and put our complete trust in You. We are Your small children, we depend on You, and we need Your strength today. Let my husband breathe peacefully during the surgery, with no threat from his recent cold.

Please help me regain my strength so that I can be my husband's best possible nurse, wife, advocate, and trusted friend. Blessed, blessed are You.

We were admitted to the pre-surgery room at 9:55 a.m. but did not see our surgeon until 2:30 p.m. We waited four hours in the freezing cubicle, my husband dressed only in a hospital gown and me in only lightweight clothing. The nurses heated cotton blankets in the microwave for us to ward off the cold. Covered in the blankets, we looked like we were in a tent. The nurses kept checking on why there was such a long delay, and one especially kind nurse gave my husband her heated, therapeutic neck collar filled with buckwheat, which helped support his neck on the uncomfortable gurney.

Turns out the 7:30 a.m. surgical slot had been taken by a man who had required seven hours of surgery, four more hours than the norm. We prayed for him and his family as well as the surgeon (praying he would be rested and fit when our time came).

Despite the cold we filled the hours with very special, quiet bonding time. I had the chance to lie next to my husband, pray over him, kiss and hug him, massage him, and reminisce about our life together—all the things I wanted to do last night but was too tired to do.

When our surgeon finally peeked his head into our cubicle, he said our surgery would be at 3:30 p.m. and that he would make every attempt to save the nerve bundles that pass through the prostate, to ensure erectile functioning and bladder control: "According to the sexual functioning questionnaire you filled out in my office, I know this is important to you." Before he left I gave him a hug and said I wanted to bless him. He graciously accepted.

When the surgery began I called everyone and told them the surgery had been delayed, and that I would call them in five hours with an update. Then I returned to the car, called Silent Unity to ask them to pray, and ate my breakfast/lunch/dinner. For the next five hours I prayed, walked around the beautiful grounds at City of Hope, read, and waited.

City of Hope has a beautiful multi-acre campus, carefully designed to assist the healing process. There are majestic tall trees; a rose garden filled with every shade of color; sculptures of children, families, animals, and religious figures; benches scattered on the lush lawns; the most exquisite Japanese garden—filled with Japanese structures, a koi pond with multicolored koi, turtles, and cat fish; and beautiful Japanese landscaping—bamboo, granite rocks, lily pads. There are little cottages for families from out of town whose loved ones are there for long-term treatments.

5:30 p.m.—I got a call from the surgical nurse saying, "Everything is going fine. The doctor says he should be finished in one hour." This was really reassuring news!

6:30 p.m.—The surgeon phoned me in the waiting area and said:

"Your husband's operation went so nicely. He did beautifully with the anesthesia. There was minimal bleeding. His prostate was nice and smooth. Some of the lymph nodes were slightly enlarged, but none of them were discolored. I was able to save his left nerve bundle and some

of the right bundle. He had a penile erection as he woke up. I also removed the seminal vesicles. Everything will be sent to the lab and we will have a pathology report in four to five days."

8:30 p.m.—My husband was transferred to his private room. He was groggy from the anesthesia and looked very fragile. It was a big operation, and it had taken a lot out of him. His sense of humor was there, however. When the nurse asked him his name and his date of birth, he gave a fictitious name. The anesthesia made him less reserved than usual, and I thought it was funny. He doesn't remember saying it. His legs were wrapped in compression hose and cuffs, which prevent blood clots. I saw the Foley catheter and felt sorry for him having to wear it.

Assured that he was safely settled and in good hands, I made the long drive home in the dark and arrived at 11:00 p.m. It had been a fifteen-hour day, and I was exhausted!

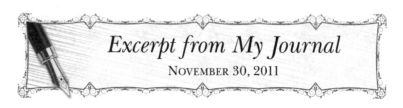

Excerpt from My Journal
November 30, 2011

I DECIDED TO SLEEP IN THIS MORNING AS THE HOSPITAL CALLED and said my husband wouldn't be ready for discharge until around 2:30 p.m. When I arrived in his room the nurse gave me a thorough demonstration and explanation about caring for the Foley catheter.

I had never really paid too much attention to the catheter when I was an oncology social worker. It was something the older men had in the hospital. I never asked them about the impact of having one. Now, because it was my husband—who, prior to the surgery, was in robust health, and who is pretty young— I looked at it in an entirely different light. I knew the catheter was a huge blow to his ego, and he told me it was very uncomfortable. As I watched the demonstration about how to take care of it I became anxious, afraid I might make a mistake. As the wife I would be doing the twenty-four-hour care for seven straight days. (In the hospital the nurses are on shifts that last eight, ten, or twelve hours; then they are relieved.) In addition, I would be monitoring the healing of his incisions and looking out for any complications to his recovery.

I would say we were both pretty nervous on the long ride home from the hospital. I tried to be cheery and encouraging: "We can do this. We've been through your partial hip replacement. We'll take our time and you will heal."

Recovery from this major surgery, however, was very difficult for both of us. It was quite different than any prior surgery. My husband was in a great deal of pain at the incision sites, in his abdomen, and in his rectum. When the prostate, lymph nodes, and seminal vesicles are removed, the bladder and the rectum become inflamed and sore because they are adjacent to the prostate. The urethra passes through the prostate and has to be cut when the prostate is removed. At the end of the sur-

gery it has to be reconnected to the mouth of the bladder. A catheter is used while the bladder and urethra heal.

A catheter is a plastic tube that is inserted into the penis, with a balloon that is inflated once it is inside the bladder to keep it from falling out. There is some movement of the catheter when the man shifts his position, even though the tube is taped to the groin area. This movement causes irritation, some bleeding, and pain to any scar tissue in the penis that resulted from the surgery.

The catheter is attached to a large plastic bag, which collects the urine. The urine has to be measured, inspected for blood, and emptied before it overflows. The bag has to be held in a position that is lower than the bladder so that the urine can drain properly. This can be done by draping the bag over a bed rail or chair at the bedside, or by the man holding it as he walks, which is really awkward and embarrassing. The other option is to change to a smaller bag, which can be taped to the man's leg. To accommodate the bag the man must wear loose-fitting pants, shorts, or a long night shirt.

My husband said the catheter was more difficult to deal with than the actual surgery. He hated it. It was painful, interfered with his sleeping, and was inconvenient. In the morning and evening we had to wash off the blood that had hardened on the tube of the catheter and retracted into the penis, and we had to put Lidocaine around the tip of the irritated penis.

From a psychological point of view, a man's penis represents his manhood, his virility, his self-image, his sexuality. Prostate cancer strikes at the very heart of the man's vulnerability. This organ, which is supposed to be strong, hard, and potent, is rendered dysfunctional and incontinent after prostate surgery—a scenario that can last at least two months and sometimes forever. These two conditions can be devastating. It saddens me to see my husband going through this.

Another problem he experienced was a great deal of pain in the rectum. We had not been told to expect it. He felt the discomfort only when he was sitting. He experimented with sitting on a pillow and a donut-ring pillow. We tried hot showers, but the pain is internal. Nothing really helped.

The combination of the catheter and the pain in the abdomen, penis, and rectum made my husband very disinclined to walk around the house for a half-hour per day, as the doctor had recommended. He did not want to walk. I pushed him to walk laps around the house. Our dog and I walked with him. We argued about walking. I had to back off. It was his body.

In terms of food, the dietician gave my husband instructions about what he was supposed to eat: soft, bland diet the first few days followed by gradual inclusion of solid food. I tried to incorporate some of the anti-cancer foods, which he resisted. He got angry with me: "I want to eat what I normally eat. I don't like these changes. My life has changed. Things have been taken away from me. You have to let me eat what I want."

I understood his anger, his frustration, his recent losses, and the pain. It was normal for him to be angry. He wanted his life to be like it used to be prior to the cancer. He wanted to be in control of his life. I tried not to take it personally, but it did hurt. I was trying hard to help him fight the cancer. I wanted him to live. I was tired. My life had been turned upside down too. Even our dog knew something was wrong; he sensed that my husband was fragile, and he was very careful not to bump into him or bark. He knew Daddy was not doing well.

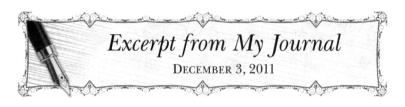

Excerpt from My Journal

DECEMBER 3, 2011

SHEER AND UTTER EXHAUSTION OF BODY, MIND, EMOTIONS, *and spirit. My husband and I feel like we have been hit by a series of trucks. We went to bed at 8:30 p.m.*

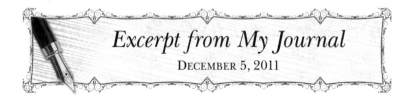

Excerpt from My Journal

DECEMBER 5, 2011

I AWOKE REFRESHED. I WALKED BRUTIE, MADE AN EARLY BREAKFAST, assisted my husband with a shower, and worked on paying bills. I had a therapy session with a client whose dog had been put to sleep the previous week. We both had a good cry and shared precious memories of the dog. Because of my experience with the cancer I was especially sensitive to my client's loss and sadness.

I made lunch and bought some unscented natural laundry detergent and beautiful fresh salmon.

I made dinner—salad, salmon, lentil/chicken broth soup. Both my husband and I had big appetites. We watched a rental movie and went to bed early.

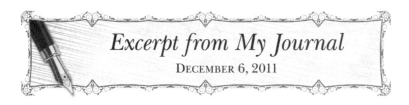

Excerpt from My Journal
DECEMBER 6, 2011

DEAREST LORD,

Today is exactly one week since my husband's surgery. We are going to City of Hope tomorrow to have the catheter removed. How do they deflate the balloon inside the bladder and retract the plastic tube from the penis? Won't that be terribly painful?

My husband is becoming depressed and silently terrified about hearing the results of the surgical pathology report. Of course it is frightening! That report is going to have a HUGE EFFECT on the next phase of our lives.

I went to the drugstore to buy some incontinence pads. We were told to expect some leakage when the catheter is removed. This "temporary incontinence" can last six weeks or longer. The urethra was cut in order to remove the prostate, so it takes some time to heal. In addition, my husband lost some of the nerves that assisted in bladder control. He is to practice Kegel exer-

cises, which strengthen the urinary sphincter muscle and the pelvic floor muscles, which in turn will assist in re-establishing continence and erectile functioning.

We pray with all our hearts that the cancer was contained inside the prostate capsule, that none escaped to surrounding or distant parts. Please let there be no more cancer. Let it be gone.

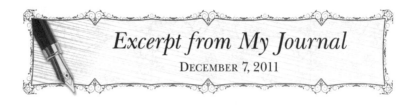

Excerpt from My Journal
DECEMBER 7, 2011

DEAREST LORD,

Here we are at City of Hope. My husband had a blood test, and now we are waiting to see the surgeon. His nurse did a really nice job of removing the catheter. She described every step of what she was doing to ease my husband's fear and dread: "First I will deflate the balloon inside. Next, take a very deep breath and hold it. When I tell you to exhale I will have quickly and painlessly removed it."

The surgeon finally walked in and explained the surgical pathology report: "I am afraid some of the cancer grew outside the capsule and moved into the right seminal vesicle. Some more of the cancer grew right up to the margin of the capsule."

We were silent and wide-eyed. He continued: "The lymph nodes were all negative for cancer." I quickly said, "Well, that's *really good news, isn't it? If it's not in the lymph nodes there is less chance of metastasis." The surgeon responded: "One is not better than the other. With the invasion into the seminal vesicle there is a higher risk for cancer recurrence, as it may shed cells into the bloodstream."*

Then he described the surgery: "I removed the prostate, the seminal vesicles on the right and left side, and the pelvic lymph nodes. I removed some of the right bundle of nerves but was able to leave all of the left bundle."

Now my husband spoke: "If you were able to leave some of the nerves, does that mean I will regain my continence?" The surgeon replied: "Don't worry about the unknown. You can regain bladder control by practicing the Kegel exercises three times a day. In the beginning, just do one set of ten each time. Gradually you can increase the reps. You have to squeeze the muscles in your lower abdomen and hold them for a count of five seconds, then release. Try doing them as you urinate. Pee, then stop the flow of urine, then pee again. Build the muscle stamina gradually."

Then my husband asked, "Were you able to remove all of the cancer?" The surgeon replied: "As far as I know. I feel pretty confident. But there is always a chance that there are some microtumors somewhere in your body. The bottom line is that we will appraise your progress all along. You will come back for your first post-surgery PSA test in one month. It is not necessary or prudent to do something right now, like radiation. If you have radiation too soon after surgery it can impair your bladder control forever." We asked if we could travel to our home in Santa Fe, New Mexico, for Christmas and he said it would be fine and probably good for us.

The surgeon gave my husband a prescription for Viagra, explaining: "Even though you currently have ED, research shows that Viagra stimulates the flow of blood to the penis and can help in the healing process and restoring sexual functioning. You will take 50 mg a day for nine months. My nurse will phone the order to your pharmacy." This news gave my husband and I some hope that he might regain his erectile functioning.

On the way home the two of us had a lot to talk about. My husband said, "I am confident that all the cancer was removed." With the type of Grade 5 cancer cells he had, I told him I hoped and prayed it was true but that I was not so sure: "I don't trust the cancer." He was wearing his incontinence pad in his underwear, and I was making the long drive in rush-hour traffic. By the time we got home the pad was soaking wet. We ate a small dinner and went to bed.

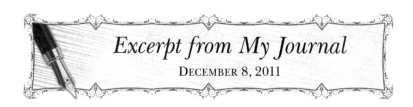

Excerpt from My Journal
DECEMBER 8, 2011

WHEN WE WOKE UP TODAY WE REALIZED THE SURGEON HAD not given us a copy of the surgical pathology report. We called his nurse practitioner and requested one. After running into some resistance from the medical records department she was finally able to secure a copy and email it to us. When we read it I was overjoyed to see that the pathologist had downgraded the Gleason score to 7 (4+3, with tertiary pattern of 5):

SURGICAL PATHOLOGY REPORT

Prostatic Adenocarcinoma. Primary Gleason Pattern: Grade 4. Secondary Gleason Pattern: Grade 3. Tertiary Gleason Pattern: Grade 5. Of the lymph nodes, 3 right pelvic lymph nodes were negative for metastatic carcinoma. 4 left pelvic lymph nodes were also negative. Tumor is present in both left and right sides of the prostate and involves approximately 17% of the tissue submitted for examination. Tumor is present in extraprostatic soft tissue, left and right posterior. Tumor is present in right seminal vesicle. Tumor is present at the soft tissue resection margin.

After we read the report and talked about it we were grateful for the lower Gleason score. It gave us hope that the cancer was not as dangerous as the surgeon had suggested. We needed to have some hope.

Dearest Lord, we did not get a "perfect score" on the pathology report. Our prayers that the cancer would be confined to the prostate capsule did not come true. Help us to accept what we cannot change and have the courage to do what we can to fight and conquer the cancer. Please help us with this next phase— waiting to see what the PSA number will be.

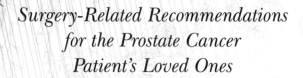

*Surgery-Related Recommendations
for the Prostate Cancer
Patient's Loved Ones*

1. On the day of the surgery you will be in the hospital for many hours. I recommend that you **pack a number of items in your car for your own self-care**: bottled water, Thermos of warm beverage, nutritious food, books to read, and layers of warm clothing for you and your patient (as hospitals, especially surgery and recovery areas, are notoriously cold). When there are delays in the schedule you do not want to be freezing, which will add to your stress.

2. **Be very careful to wash your hands with soap and warm water when you go to the bathroom.** There are many airborne germs in a hospital. Try to avoid touching your eyes, nose, and mouth with your hands.

3. **When you are waiting, spend some time walking outdoors.** Hospitals can be gloomy and sterile environments. Nature will boost your mood, and walking will circulate your blood and ease tension.

4. **Pray for your patient and for the surgical and recovery staff.** Surgeons and their staffs work long hours, dedicated to saving lives. They themselves are under a lot of stress, fatigue, and pressure. Your prayers will give them energy and guide their hands in the care of your loved one.

5. **Arrange to have a support team**, available in person or by phone, to assist you and your loved one. Don't go through this alone.

6. **Acknowledge your fear and apprehension**— normal emotions when your loved one is going to have major surgery. Shift the focus of your emotions from fear to love and hope by practicing relaxed breathing and meditations with positive outcomes.

7. **Try to get some rest.** When your patient is discharged from the hospital, the hard work begins. If you have children, arrange child care so you can focus on your patient and yourself. When you're in the role of caregiver you will experience an increase in fatigue. It's a lot of responsibility to be the twenty-four-hour nurse at home.

   You will also tend to carry your patient's emotions on your own shoulders in an effort to help him in his recovery from surgery. This will only add to your fatigue.

Give yourself permission to be less concerned with running a "perfect looking" home and just try to cover the basics for now. If someone offers to help with house care and meals, accept the help with humility and gratitude.

Dear loved one of the prostate cancer patient, I have written this special meditation for you. I suggest you read it daily:

In this time of stress and uncertainty I surrender my need to be in control, and I trust that my loved one will have a successful outcome.

I acknowledge my emotions and the reactions in my body, but I do not let them control me. Instead I practice deep abdominal breathing and release tension as I exhale deeply. I feel myself letting go of fear, doubt, worry, uncertainty, and anxiety. I visualize them drifting away from my body and mind.

I remind myself that, throughout my life, I have struggled with challenges and have survived to this point. I believe that strength, resiliency, and courage reside within me on the deepest level. I claim these qualities in myself.

I will stay focused on today and trust that I can get through tomorrow. I will take care of my body, mind, emotions, and spirit. I am a beautiful and valuable creation of God, and I love myself.

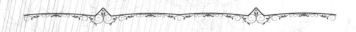

Surgery-Related Recommendations for the Prostate Cancer Patient

1. **Acknowledge your fear and apprehension.** Again, these are normal emotions when it comes to having major surgery. Shift the focus of your emotions from fear to love and hope by practicing relaxed breathing and meditations with positive outcomes.

2. **If your surgical pathology report ultimately turns out not to be what you expected, try not to be too distraught or panic.** There are many additional treatment choices that are both viable and effective. Stay in the moment. Concentrate all your efforts on healing from your surgery.

Of course we were disappointed by my husband's surgical pathology report. We had desperately wanted the cancer to be confined to the prostate capsule. To hear that it had spread to the right seminal vesicle was disheartening. We didn't yet know how serious this was or what we were going to do about it. On the other hand, we were thankful the cancer had not spread to the pelvic lymph nodes. We tried to "stay in the moment" and maintain a positive outlook.

3. **Don't be too discouraged by the catheter.** As my husband told me, it *is* inconvenient and painful and humiliating, but "this too will pass." You'll need to have it for only a week or so. It's necessary so that your bladder and urethra can heal. Take your time moving around, find comfortable positions, and keep the catheter clean to avoid infection.

When the catheter is removed you'll need to wear incontinence pads in case of leakage. Wearing pads and having "accidents" that involve wetting your bed and clothing are affronts to your sense of mastery and competence. So it's important for you and your family members to be gentle and understanding in these circumstances. It's simply a part of the process—for everyone.

MY HUSBAND'S SURGICAL PROSTATE CANCER PROFILE

GLEASON SCORE

7: *called "moderately differentiated or intermediate-grade"*

8-10: *called "poorly differentiated or high-grade"*

My husband's Gleason score:
4+3 (with tertiary pattern 5) = 7

TYPE OF CANCER

Adenocarcinoma

SURGICAL PATHOLOGY REPORT

Tumor is present in both left and right sides of the prostate

Tumor involves 17% of tissue presented for examination

Tumor is present in extraprostatic soft tissue, left and right posterior

Tumor is present at the soft tissue resection margin

PELVIC LYMPH NODES

3 right pelvic lymph nodes were negative for metastatic carcinoma

4 left pelvic lymph nodes were also negative

SEMINAL VESICLES

Tumor is present in right seminal vesicle

Another problem that may occur when the catheter is removed: a split urine stream, which is both humiliating and baffling. You may have difficulty accurately directing your urine into the toilet. It may hit the walls of the bathroom, the floor, the toilet, or your clothing. The problem stems from scar tissue in the penis or the mouth of the bladder—caused by the surgery or irritation from the catheter.

My husband experienced the split urine stream after his catheter was removed. When he visited Internet chat rooms for men recovering from prostate surgery, he found that many men were dealing with this same problem—and concluding they just had to live with it. Not true.

To correct my husband's problem, his urologist saw him in the office one day and used a surgical device to scope and then remove scar tissue from the urethra. He did not use any anesthesia. My husband said the procedure was the most pain he had ever experienced in his life, and that he had nearly passed out. As he said to the urologist: "I would never allow you to do that again without the use of anesthesia!" The urologist seemed surprised.

For the month that followed, my husband was told to use a catheter once a day at home, to prevent the return of the scar tissue. It was scary and somewhat painful, but it solved the problem.

4. **You'll experience some amount of pain in the rectum.** This, too, is a side effect of the surgery. The rectum is swollen and irritated. It needs time to heal—but the pain will diminish. Try a hot bath when your doctor clears you to do so, or sit on a soft cushion.

5. **Kegel exercises are invaluable for re-establishing your bladder functioning.** Be sure to practice them daily, as recommended. Don't be discouraged if the benefits aren't immediate as it can take six to twelve weeks to see results. Your bladder and urethra need time to heal. Your urinary sphincter muscle and pelvic floor muscles need time to strengthen. According to the website *www.kegel-exercises.com*, the pelvic muscles are found in a hammock-like structure between the urinary and anal sphincters. The pelvic floor muscles keep the bladder valve shut.

This wonderful website features diagrams of the locations of these muscles, along with audio and video directions, PDF files, and detailed explanations. Unfortunately, surgeons and urologists tend not to go into enough detail about these wonderful exercises, which were developed by Dr. Arnold Kegel. The medical establishment just says "do them" without giving men the proper information and resources. If men were consistently told that Kegel exercises can re-establish bladder control and enhance sexual functioning, they would be much more moti-vated to do them. In my experience as a psychotherapist, men do very well with concrete explanations and instructions. They like to know **why** they are doing something, and they want step-by-step instructions on **how** to do it. Websites like *www.kegel-exercises.com* fit the bill on both counts.

Right after surgery, my husband was able to hold the muscles for only three seconds at a time, with a five-second rest in between. As I am writing this nine months later, he is able to hold the mus-cles for fifteen seconds. He has developed his own "workout routine" for the Kegel exercises, which he does twice a day, morning and evening: nine repetitions, holding the muscles for fifteen seconds, with a five-second rest in between. After that he does twelve quick squeeze/releases. This routine has helped him regain 95 percent of his continence to date.

Kegel exercises, by the way, also help women with both post-child-delivery incontinence and stress incontinence.

6. **Understand that anger is a normal reaction to losing control.** With this type of surgery your body is invaded by the surgical team, you have to stay in the hospital, and you temporarily lose control of your erections and continence. It's a lot of change and loss. You also experience considerable pain, which makes you even grouchier. Acknowledge your anger, but try not to direct it toward your loved ones personally. They love you, after all, and they're trying to help you. Try to express your anger directly: "I am really angry with this cancer. I don't like losing control. I don't like the changes in my body. I am embarrassed by my lack of sexual functioning and incontinence."

Besides the anger, try to express the vulnerable feelings underneath: "I'm afraid of so many things. Will I regain my sexual functioning and continence? Will this pain ever go away? What will the surgical pathology report reveal? What's going to happen to us? Will you still love me if I have to wear incontinence pads and cannot have an erection? How are people going to treat me if they find out I have cancer?"

Dear prostate cancer patient, I have written this special meditation for you. I suggest you read it daily:

This is a challenging period for me. I take a moment to reflect on events in my past that challenged me but that I overcame with determination, belief in myself, and creative solutions. I savor the strength and resiliency that reside within me. **I am a warrior**, *a survivor.*

As a man, my masculinity and value are not determined by the functioning of my body parts. Temporary erectile dysfunction and incontinence do not define me or make me inadequate. I take this opportunity to turn within and invite the Universe to help me grow in new ways. My self-confidence and self-esteem remain intact.

I am a blessed creation of God, a husband/lover, father, grandfather, friend, mentor, neighbor, worker or boss. I have integrity, talent, and worth. I trust in my body's ability to search out and destroy the cancer. I will be gentle and accepting of my body as it is healing. I love myself and give love and forgiveness to the people in my life. I await the future with positive expectations and maintain practices that ensure peacefulness.

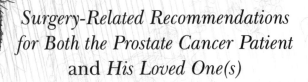

Surgery-Related Recommendations for Both the Prostate Cancer Patient and *His Loved One(s)*

1. **Take naps and go to bed early.** Sleep is recuperative and recharges the body, mind, emotions, and spirit.

2. **Find some ways to lighten your mood.** Movies can be fun and distracting. Music can lift your spirit. You probably won't feel like having visitors while dealing with the catheter, so find some fun activities to distract yourselves. Look for something to laugh about.

3. **Be gentle with each other and bask in the opportunity to be of service.** Love is all about actions. It's easy to tell someone you love him/her. The message is much more believable when it is seen and felt. None of us knows how long our life will be. Celebrate the moment. Embrace one another. Share your feelings and your hearts. Comfort each other with hugs and kisses. Support and understand each other. You will get through this.

4. **Incorporate anti-cancer foods into your diet.** The surgery has done its job. Now it's your turn to do something. Eat foods that will boost your

immune functioning. Give those natural killer cells the energy and nutrition they need to search out and destroy any micro tumors that may have escaped. Although you are in need of emotional comfort, try to avoid eating traditional "comfort foods": carbohydrates made of white flour and white pasta, bakery goods, pizza, fried items. Avoid sugar too as it promotes the growth of cancer cells.

5. **Engage in as much walking as you can tolerate.** Force yourself to walk at least a half-hour per day during this time of recovery. Walking helps eliminate internal fluids that accumulate during surgery. It also prevents blood clots, oxygenates the body, and releases tension. Do it! Walking is also a bonding activity for you and your loved one.

6. **Spend time outdoors and with family pets if you have them.** Nature and animals are healing and uplifting.

CHAPTER FIVE

Waiting for the First Post-Surgery PSA Results

Waiting for my husband's first post-surgery PSA test results was strange—a period of time I don't even like to remember. We had already lived through the diagnosis, the treatment decision making, the surgery, and the surgical pathology report. Now we were "in between." We would have to wait an entire month to find out if the surgery had removed all the cancer.

What were we to do with our emotions, our not knowing?

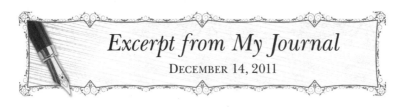

Excerpt from My Journal
December 14, 2011

Although we had wanted to be optimistic that the surgery had removed all the cancer, a meeting with the urologist popped that bubble. He was very pleased that the surgical pathology report revealed a Gleason 7 (4+3) rather than the initial Gleason 9 (4+5) from the biopsy report. He told us, however: "Don't be lulled by the Gleason score. **The fact that the cancer spread beyond the prostate capsule and into the right seminal vesicle is dangerous.** *The best hope for cure is to have radiation in that area shortly after the surgery. I recommend you meet with the radiation oncologist at St. John's Hospital when you return from Santa Fe."*

We followed his recommendation and made an appointment for January 5, 2012. By the same token we decided to keep our January 16, 2012, appointment with the surgeon at City of Hope. My husband will have his first PSA test after the surgery there, and we will discuss what City of Hope provides in the way of radiation.

Meanwhile, we have both returned to work and are planning to leave December 19 for Christmas vacation at our second home in Santa Fe. It is a two-day, nine-hundred-mile drive— through Flagstaff, Arizona and Gallup, New Mexico—and it will be very cold. We will stay the first night in Williams, Arizona. There is a lot of packing to do for the trip, and we will need to make special preparations for my husband's comfort en route as well as his incontinence.

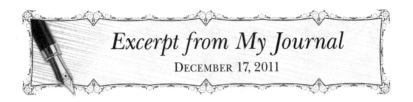

Excerpt from My Journal
DECEMBER 17, 2011

DREAM IMAGES:

"A stranger, who is threatening, has moved into our house. It has changed our lives, our dynamic, and we don't like it.

My legs have been knocked out from under me.

I have been hit by a freight train, and my body, mind, emotions, and spirit are flying through the air. I don't know where I am going to land and what shape I will be in. Will I survive? Will my various parts stack together once again, or will I be a casualty?"

Last night was the first night in nearly four weeks that we could sit on our large daybed in the family room, in our normal order, and watch television: my husband on the left, me in the middle, and Brutie on the right ... or climbing over me and sitting next to my husband, giving him kisses or laying his head into his body and receiving kisses and massage. Prior to that my husband had to sit on a separate chair next to the daybed—because he had the catheter or was too sore from his surgery.

This is also the first time in four weeks I was able to say, "I need to be the baby." My husband was able to make me a large sorbet/ice cream sundae and serve it in my tall Depression-era glass. (I use the phrase "I need to be the baby" when I am tired of being the responsible adult and need to be taken care of by my husband. In these instances he takes care of me by preparing a sundae, rubbing my feet, giving me a massage, or preparing the meal. In return he can say the same phrase, and I take care of him by preparing special recipes from his childhood, massaging him, covering him with hugs and kisses.)

I was hit by a blast of exhaustion this evening and was compelled to take a hot bath and go straight to bed. Watching television, I could not lift my head off the pillow. I was afraid to ask for a sundae for fear my husband would eat something sweet that would feed his cancer. But I was exhausted: My life had been really hard these last four weeks, I had been in the strictly adult-nurse-server role, and my Inner Child needed a treat, something sweet, to be taken care of once again by my husband.

He was very understanding, supportive, and happy to do it. In fact, I'm sure he was happy to get out of the "patient" role and return to his normal caretaker role. Brutie sensed that my husband was stronger tonight, no longer tethered to a catheter, no longer so sore in his tummy with his seven incisions, once more the Daddy to us all.

This evening brought an infusion of energy and hope back into my veins. I was tired, stripped of energy, and I very much needed to be taken care of. I am struck by another dilemma, though: We are a "foodie" family. How are we going to embrace an anti-cancer diet and maintain the satisfaction we have always gotten from food? We have so many traditions associated with food: family gatherings, dinners, going out for meals on our weekend dates, watching television. In all of these instances we have special food that we enjoy.

I want to do everything in my power to provide anti-cancer meals and treats for my husband: agave sweetener, soy creamer for his faux coffee, only wheat or multigrain bread products, nayonaise instead of mayonnaise, omega 3, free-range eggs, mainly fish and chicken for protein, heavy amounts of fruit and vegetables.

But these are changes for my husband, and he does not like many of them. I have to give him the right of self-determination. It is his body, his cancer, his destiny to control. His whole life he has loved sweets and carbohydrates. The cancer has invaded his body and his life. Doesn't he have the right to treat himself with the chips he likes; the sundaes he loves; the non-caffeine, non-sugar sodas he likes; his favorite mayonnaise for his tuna sandwiches; his occasional pizza and fries? Some red meat, pork, and lamb?

What quality of life will he have, what pleasure will he have, if this foodie cannot eat his favorite foods? I must let go and let him make his own decisions. I cannot control him even if I want to. I must surrender my will and ask God to protect and guide him in this process.

I, too, am a foodie. I eat very healthy and happen to love most of the anti-cancer foods: whole grains, quinoa, mushrooms,

Brussels sprouts, kale, leafy greens, seaweed, tofu, soy products, kefir, fruit. But even I love to eat popcorn and have a sorbet/ice cream sundae once a week, lamb, pork, occasional steak, Indian naan, Mexican food. I want to eat these foods, as always, but I want to be a responsible "food model" for my husband.

He has already been on the urologist's anti-inflammation diet for over a year, without a complaint: no caffeine, no chocolate, no alcohol, no strong spices. He has totally regulated himself, and I am very proud of him. It may, in fact, have retarded the growth of his very aggressive cancer.

Yesterday my husband sent an email to my brother, telling him that his prostate had been removed and to give us a call. This was a relief to me. I hoped it meant that I could now share this news with more members of my family. It is very hard and probably detrimental to have to keep it a secret; for in not sharing we do not receive the love and prayer support we so desperately need.

Thoughts About the Holidays

Ordinarily we look forward to driving to Santa Fe for Christmas and New Year's. We enjoy driving along Route 66 from California and through northern Arizona and New Mexico. It gives us the chance to talk, enjoy the beautiful scenery, and de-stress from city life. This year, however, we approach the holidays with fatigue and the return of SHOCK. So many dramatic things have happened in a short period of time:

11-11-11 Prostate cancer diagnosis

11-29-11 Robotic-assisted radical prostatectomy

12-7-11 Removal of the catheter and beginning of incontinence and erectile dysfunction; post-surgical pain in abdomen and rectum

12-8-11 Surgical pathology report states cancer invaded the right seminal vesicle

12-14-11 Urologist recommends radiation as next treatment

We are exhausted and numb to our emotions. I have a lot of planning to do this week as I am concerned about my husband's fragile physical state. I am worried that the long drive will exacerbate the pain in his abdomen and rectum. I go to REI and purchase an air mattress and down sleeping bag, which would allow him to lie down and keep warm for the winter drive. He has to pack loose-fitting clothing that won't hurt his incisions and that will allow him to change his incontinence pads en route.

Part of me feels too tired to make the nine-hundred-mile drive, but the other part of me wants to escape the cancer, the treatment decisions, and the uncertainty that lay ahead. I tell myself, "We need the distraction. We need some fun. We need to continue our family traditions."

My husband chose to sit in the front seat of the car the whole way. The trip was pretty uneventful except for the snowstorms, whiteout conditions, and the many times my husband had to change his pads. He never complained about his pain or his incontinence, and I greatly admire him. The long drive gave him a chance to sleep a lot and recover from the surgery.

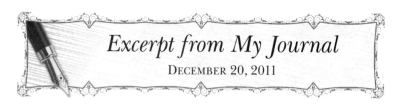

Excerpt from My Journal
December 20, 2011

When we arrived in Santa Fe our heater was not working and the room temperature inside the house was 30 degrees. It was freezing! We turned up the radiant heater but knew it would take two days to warm the floors and the entire house. Meanwhile, I made fires in the two fireplaces and added layers of down comforters to our bed. We dressed in sweaters, insulated pants, gloves, and hats. It looked like a scene out of the movie Doctor Zhivago. *In a way it was like an adventure, and it was kind of funny. We huddled in bed, drank hot soup, and watched the steam spiraling from the cups and our mouths.*

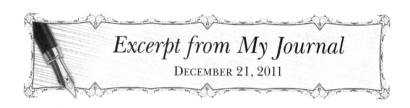

Excerpt from My Journal
December 21, 2011

It's my birthday today and the cold is no longer funny. It's just plain freezing! And people get grouchy when they are freezing. I called my contractor, and he can't get a repair man over until tomorrow. He is out of town until next week.

To make matters worse, I am very disappointed with the construction project that was supposed to be completed when we arrived. I have been building a minka—*a small version of a two-hundred-year-old Japanese farmhouse—in my backyard for the last two years. The first year consisted of putting up the massive eight-by-eight-inch support beams of Douglas fir on a concrete foundation; building the intricate roof of eight-by-eight-inch intertwining beams and cedar decking; constructing a steel-paneled, steep-pitched roof; and building one stucco wall that contains the electrical outlets. I had studied Japanese architectural books for two years before coming up with my design. This was the dream of a lifetime.*

The second year of the project involved closing in the minka with three more stucco walls and specially designed, custom sliding shoji window panels and massive shoji doors, made from Spanish cedar. I had waited four months to see my windows and doors. You have no idea how excited I was to see the completion of this project. This was to be my "spiritual space and refuge," and I so needed it right now.

When I first saw my windows and doors I thought they were absolutely gorgeous. On closer inspection, however, I realized that there were major mechanical and design flaws. The sliding elements of the windows and doors had been mounted on the outside track, in direct pathway of the snow and ice. To make matters worse, they were placed on wooden tracks, with-

out any rollers, which made them nearly impossible to move. In fact, one day they were frozen shut, and I had to use a hair dryer to thaw the ice so I could move them—using two hands and a shoulder leaning into them.

Compounding the problem, the tracks were designed with a half-inch space between the glass panels, which allowed the wind and snow to blow into the minka. I had to stuff crumpled newspapers in between the gaps, and these windows are five by five feet and the doors are five by eight feet! I called the contractor's foreman to come over and complained to him that there were "design and installation flaws," and that I was very unhappy. He said he thought there was nothing that could be done: "To pull out the windows and doors with the hope of reinstalling them in the proper order would destroy them."

The icing on the cake was that the brand new cast-iron, wood-burning stove had a crack along its base and could not be used. I had to go to the hardware store to see if another one was available, call the foreman to disconnect my stove, return it to the store, and pick up and install the second stove.

On the way home I stopped at a favorite restaurant and picked up dinner. By the time I got home I was exhausted and totally depressed. "So much for spending my birthday in my beloved minka," I told myself. This was the most disappointing of birthdays!

My husband tried to lift my mood by giving me a birthday card. The card was sweet, but I went to bed depressed.

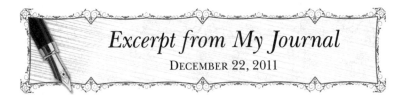

Excerpt from My Journal
DECEMBER 22, 2011

I WAKE UP FEELING DEPRESSED. I CAN'T BELIEVE THAT THE CON-tractor, his foreman, and the owner of the window and door company would install the windows and doors and NOT NOTICE there is a problem!

This is northern New Mexico, which is frigid in the winter with heavy winds and snow, and which has heavy winds and monsoon rain in the summer. What were these guys thinking? Why didn't they notice the problem and call me about it?

I discussed the problem with my husband today and was shocked and overwhelmed when he told me: "Shame on you for not being on top of it. You should have been specific in your design, in the mechanics. It's your project."

His response floored me. This is my supportive husband? This is the man I have been taking care of for the last month and a half? That I have placed my life on hold for and made my top priority? This is how he honors me? He shames me and tells me I, a lay person, am supposed to know more than my contractor, his foreman, and the owner of the window and door company?

I was so depressed and broken-hearted at that point that I got up from the breakfast table and went into the closet in our bedroom. I crouched in the corner, my arms wrapped around my knees, and began sobbing like a baby. I could not move.

My husband got worried after twenty minutes and walked around the house, searching for me. He tiptoed into the bathroom and moved toward the walk-in closet. When he saw me on the floor, in the corner, he quietly turned around, walked back into the kitchen, and returned with a hot cup of coffee, which he offered me. He told Brutie, who followed him, "Mommy needs to be quiet for a little while." Brutie came up to me, licked my tears, and sat quietly beside me.

With the coffee and the kindness he had shown me, I was able to rejoin my husband. We had a long talk about the problems with the minka, and he said he would help me in whatever way he could. We would have to meet with the contractor next week and determine if there could be a solution. The contractor might walk away, since he had been paid. Even if he were willing to make changes it might be very expensive. The bottom line was that we would work together as a team.

My husband told me later that it broke his heart to see me so despondent. I realized that because of the cancer and his painful recovery, he had not wanted to get involved and was a bit irritated that there was a problem. Normally he would not shame me. I was able to forgive him and gratefully accepted his help and counsel. With his background in engineering he figured out that the tracks for the windows and doors needed to be steel or aluminum over the wood sill, with rollers, to allow for easy sliding. He also recommended that the frames for the windows and doors be dovetailed so that they would fit tightly.

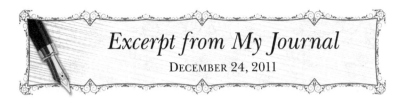

Excerpt from My Journal
DECEMBER 24, 2011

IN RETROSPECT I CAN SEE THAT GOD ALLOWED THESE PROBLEMS with the minka as a distraction from the cancer. We forgot about the cancer and spent days working as a team to solve the problems. As usual we had fun working together. We love to discuss things and situations. We talked about the approaching meeting with the contractor, anticipated what he would say, what we would say. My husband was in his helper/problem solver role. I was benefiting from his help. Our love and respect for one another was rekindled.

I felt so encouraged today that I went into town and bought a small artificial Christmas tree, lights, and handmade New Mexican- and Native American-style ornaments for a surprise Christmas morning in the minka. My husband surprised me by making dinner reservations at La Fonda Hotel for a belated birthday dinner. My joy has returned, and this was a very good day!

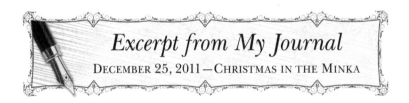

Excerpt from My Journal
DECEMBER 25, 2011 — CHRISTMAS IN THE MINKA

I GOT UP EARLY AND WENT OUT TO THE MINKA. THE SUN WAS shining and it was a wee bit warmer. I started a fire in the woodburning stove, played Christmas music, and treated myself to a yoga session on the tatami mat platform. Brutie sat on the platform beside me, and I made a video recording. What a beautiful way to celebrate Christmas, doing yoga and listening to Celine Dion singing Christmas carols. My husband was still in bed. I was dressed in insulated pants, a turtleneck, a wool Norwegian sweater, and a Russian-style lambskin hat.

I walked back into the house, woke up my husband with a Christmas kiss, and told him to dress warmly in a jacket, insulated pants, and his Russian-style hat and gloves. I ushered him out to the minka to see the tree and the lights, and had him sit on the couch next to the wood stove while I went inside to prepare a special Christmas breakfast. When it was ready I set up Japanese lacquer trays with the food and hot drinks. We sat in Japanese-style chairs, covered with Pendleton wool blankets. We took pictures and laughed about how funny we looked: hot air steaming from our mouths and our drinks, shivering in the cold.

My husband gave me a Christmas card he had made. Because of the surgery and recovery he had been unable to buy me a present. He made the card with an envelope decorated by the words "Peace," "Love," "Joy," "Joyeux Noel." It was the most beautiful, wonderful, special Christmas morning we have ever had! It did not matter in the least that we hadn't been able to buy each other presents. Love, joy, and life were the best presents ever. We were very grateful.

Later that day we went to the fabulous Christmas Day buffet at La Fonda Hotel, as was our yearly custom. We were happy to join the happy crowd and were amazed, as always, to see the buffet table spread with every possible delicacy and ice sculptures. We gave ourselves permission to eat anything we wanted—red meat and dessert included.

We asked a tourist to take a photo of us in front of the large Christmas tree in the center of the lobby. We used that photo for our yearly holiday card. Happy as we were on the inside, the picture looked pretty grim. Both of our faces showed the toll the cancer had taken. We looked exhausted and worn out, and we were.

I am happy to say that the rest of our vacation in Santa Fe was very peaceful. We met with the contractor, the foreman, and the owner of the window and door company, and they agreed to do whatever it took to solve the problems with the windows and doors.

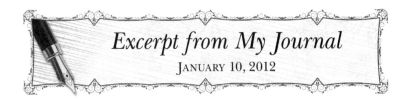

Excerpt from My Journal
JANUARY 10, 2012

DEAREST LORD,

The only way I can make it through this day is to acknowledge where and how I really am. I am depressed, Lord. I have the classic symptoms:

✦ *fatigue*

✦ *indecisiveness*

✦ *lack of enthusiasm*

✦ *feeling overwhelmed*

✦ *lack of joy*

✦ *immobility*

✦ *difficulty doing simple things*

✦ *loss of identity*

The scripture that comes to mind is: "My strength is made known in your weakness." Dearest Lord, I need Your strength, guidance, and grace. I can't seem to get a proper footing, and my spiritual and emotional stamina are lacking. Can you please help me, lift me, and carry me along?

The same two circumstances that so debilitated me in Santa Fe—the problems with the minka doors and windows along with my husband's prostate cancer—have not abated. They are the same. As such, they are robbing me of my stamina.

I am trying to be strong for my husband first and foremost, but right now I am weak. I need You desperately. My whole family of children and grandchildren are coming this weekend for a party, and I want to be joyful and celebratory.

Please help me prepare the house and make decisions about the food. I want it to be fun, easy, and comfortable for everyone. Blessed are You.

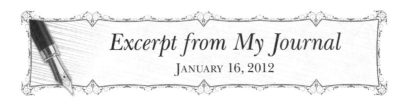

Excerpt from My Journal
JANUARY 16, 2012

*WE WENT TO CITY OF HOPE TODAY FOR MY HUSBAND'S FIRST PSA test since his surgery. After the blood was drawn we went to meet with the surgeon. When he came into the room I asked if he would sit down to talk to us: "You always seem like you're in a hurry, and we have questions to ask you." "I am in a hurry," he responded—and he remained standing. He told us: "**Your PSA score was 2.36.** There is still some cancer in your body."*

We were stunned and temporarily speechless. We were hoping that the surgeon had removed all the cancer, that the PSA would be undetectable or less than 1. When I regained my voice I said: "This is bad news, but wasn't the surgical Gleason score of 7 (4+3, with tertiary 5) a good thing?"

We were totally unprepared for the surgeon's response: "It doesn't matter if your Gleason score has 4's and 3's. Throw out the 4, throw out the 3. The fact that you have some 5's indicates you have the most aggressive, dangerous cancer cells."

He started to walk out of the room. I stopped him and asked, "So what do you recommend as the next course of treatment?" He said, "Usually radiation therapy and some sort of hormone deprivation therapy." I asked, "Are you going to set that up?" He said, "No. You have to request a consultation with the radiation oncology department. See my scheduling nurse." Then he walked out.

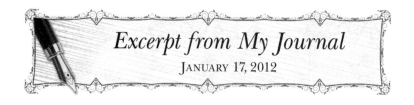

Excerpt from My Journal
JANUARY 17, 2012

DEAREST LORD, THE **PSA SCORE OF 2.36 IS SCARY INFORMA-tion!** *It is a number I was praying not to hear. I prayed for a zero or less than 1. It's good that we are seeing the urologist in two days to discuss the PSA and treatment options. We met with the radiation oncologist at St. John's on January 5, 2012, and he recommended radiation therapy and a short round of hormone deprivation therapy prior to the radiation.*

After discussing it my husband and I have already decided to do the combination of hormone deprivation therapy and radiation. We have a radiation oncology consultation scheduled with City of Hope in one week.

Lord, please, please help us. **We are fighting this cancer as hard as we can and need some positive reinforcement.** *Please bless my husband today. I know he is in shock and very discouraged. Help me to stay grounded and strong for him. Please help us to win the battle. We are Your children, and we need You. Send Your Spirit to lift us up and carry us. Send Your power to heal my husband's body and empower his natural killer cells to kill the cancer, wherever it may be growing in his body. Guide our steps, Lord.*

Thank You for directing me to Psalm 116, 1-13:

"I love the Lord because He hears my prayers and answers them. Because He bends down and listens, I will pray as long as I breathe! Death stared me in the face—I was frightened and sad. Then I cried, 'Lord, save me!'

The Lord protects the simple and the childlike. I was facing death and then He saved me. Now I can relax. For the Lord has done this wonderful miracle for me. He has saved me from death, my eyes from tears, my feet from stumbling. I shall live!"

Along-the-Journey Recommendations for the Prostate Cancer Patient and His Loved Ones

1. No matter your initial optimism, faith, hope, resolve, and hard work, **you will eventually be tested by the cancer.** There will be days when you cry, days when you fight with each other, days when you are depressed and want to give up. Some days you will be immobilized.

   There's a difference between a temporary depressed state, which lasts for a day, and *clinical depressions,* which last longer and are more debilitating. In layman's terms, here are descriptions of two different kinds of clinical depression:

Mild Depression

Feeling depressed most of the day with the following symptoms:

+ Eating too little or too much
+ Sleeping too little or too much
+ Loss of energy
+ Feeling bad about yourself
+ Being indecisive
+ Experiencing loss of hope

Usually this level of depression will not go away on its own. Outpatient psychotherapy, without the need for medication, will generally be sufficient as the treatment.

Severe Depression

Depressed mood most of the day, particularly in the morning, and a loss of interest in normal activities and relationships, with symptoms that include:

+ Your body feeling agitated, or slow and hard to move around
+ Sleeping too little or too much
+ Significant weight gain or weight loss

+ Extreme fatigue
+ Lack of motivation to do even simple tasks
+ Difficulty concentrating
+ Feeling worthless
+ Feelings of despair and hopelessness
+ Thoughts of death or suicide

As its name implies, this level of depression is severe. It will not go away by itself; it requires the combination of antidepressant medication (best prescribed by a psychiatrist, not a general practitioner) and psychotherapy. Sometimes hospitalization is required.

It's critical for you to assess the level of any depression you or your loved one(s) are experiencing. You need to help each other here. When you are depressed it may be hard for you to notice your own depression. Therefore, give each other feedback, and seek professional help when it is indicated.

Left untreated, a severe depression will rob your immune system of optimal functioning and disrupt your family and personal dynamics. It could even lead to suicide. If you seek an evaluation from a psychiatrist or begin treatment with a psychotherapist, make sure there is a coordination of treatments between your medical and psychiatric teams, which will require you to sign a release of information for one doctor to share information with another.

2. **Be kind to one another when you fight.** Most often the fight is not about the issue at hand; it is about the cancer and your helplessness, your fear, your fatigue, your disappointment, being out of control. Take time apart to assess what just happened. Try to understand the other person and what might be going on with him/her. Get back together and talk about your feelings. Forgive one another and make up.

3. **When you're in an "in-between" period— between treatments or test results—try to distract yourselves with fun activities.** Savor each day and each other as special gifts. Enjoy being alive, and live life to the fullest.

4. **Don't be afraid of the roller coaster of emotions.** They go with the territory of living with cancer. The emotions are normal reactions. You are not going crazy, and you are not a bad person. Share your emotions with one another, and find a therapist if you feel overwhelmed.

Let me say it once again: Most surgeons, urologists, radiation oncologists, and medical oncologists do not address your emotional reactions. Most of them do not refer you for pastoral counseling or psychotherapy.

On a related note, members of your extended family and your friends generally won't understand what you're going through if they haven't had cancer themselves. After the initial support they might offer at the point of diagnosis, they often become busy with their own lives and problems. Some will be uncomfortable if you discuss your roller coaster of emotions; your cancer can remind them of their own mortality and fears of dying or losing a loved one.

If you are fortunate enough to have family and friends who want to support you throughout the journey, you are indeed fortunate—and you should embrace these kind souls with open arms. It can make a world of difference.

Support groups for patients and family members can be very helpful, as can online chat groups for men with prostate cancer. The members of these groups are on the same journey and thus understand what you are going through. They offer suggestions from their own experiences, a sense of humor, and fellowship.

A word of caution, however: Even though the online chat groups for men with prostate cancer can be helpful, they can also be discouraging. My husband, for instance, went online to one of these groups. It was for men who had undergone robotic-assisted radical prostatectomy. Most of these men reported having an undetectable level of PSA after surgery. When my husband entered his PSA test results, many of the men told him, "Your surgery was a failure." This made him very discouraged—and he never returned to that particular website.

5. **Continue to engage in stress-reducing activities:** exercise, meditation, prayer, journaling, music, body massage, hot baths, excursions into nature, movies, hobbies, time with your children and grandchildren, and time with your pets and friends.

6. **Be kind and gentle with yourself.** Don't try to be perfect. Allow yourself to be weak, and admit it when you're feeling that way. Forgive yourself when you make mistakes. Ask for forgiveness. Get plenty of rest. Eat healthy foods that nour-

ish your body and support your immune system. Love yourself, and ask for TLC (tender loving care) when you need it.

7. **Practice the Serenity Prayer:** "God, grant me the serenity to accept the things I cannot change, the courage to change the things I can, and the wisdom to know the difference."

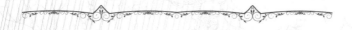

Along-the-Journey Recommendations for Doctors and Medical Staff Treating the Prostate Cancer Patient (and Helping His Loved Ones)

We prostate cancer patients and family members are able to receive disheartening news from you. It may be hard for us to grasp in the moment, and we may ask you a lot of questions, but please try to understand that **we are trying to find HOPE** and the silver lining in what you have said. We would appreciate it if you would sit down, even for a moment, and connect with us human to human, beyond just delivering the technical information. We need a kind, respectful voice, an understanding of our vulnerability, and guidance toward the next treatment. The way you treat us affects our immune systems and our ability to fight the cancer.

CHAPTER SIX

Androgen Deprivation Therapy and Radiation

WE LOST THE FIRST ROUND IN THE FIGHT TO DESTROY THE cancer; surgery had not removed all of it. Now we were at another fork in the road: We had to make a second treatment decision. What were we to do?

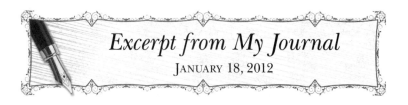

Excerpt from My Journal
JANUARY 18, 2012

THERE IS A HUGE DILEMMA WHEN DEALING WITH AN AGGRESsive form of prostate cancer: It's impossible to stay in the moment when you are constantly faced with having to make new treatment decisions based on the results of new clinical evidence. And there is added pressure because the decisions you make can save your life.

The first post-surgery PSA test result of 2.36 indicated that the cancer was still in my husband's body. The fear returned to our lives. We would have to meet with various doctors— urologist, radiation oncologists, and medical oncologists—and evaluate their recommendations. We would have to do more research in the literature. And we would have to make a decision in a short amount of time. The pressure was on.

We were faced with a series of questions:

+ *Do we elect "salvage" radiation alone? (This is radiation that follows surgery.)*

+ *Do we elect a short course of androgen deprivation therapy (ADT) with EBRT (External Beam Radiation Therapy)?*

+ *Do we elect a two-year course of androgen deprivation therapy (ADT) and radiation?*

+ *What do you do when your urologist and potential radiation oncologist at St. John's Hospital disagree? The urologist first suggested only radiation therapy. The radiation oncologist suggested a short course of ADT prior to radiation. The urologist then suggested radiation therapy and a two-year course of ADT.*

+ *What about the potential harmful side effects of ADT (osteoporosis and fractures caused by bone mineral loss, heart problems, diabetes, erectile dysfunction, loss of libido, loss of muscle strength, joint aches and pains, hot flashes, breast tenderness and growth, fatigue, changes in metabolism and body composition, depression)—or of radiation therapy (incontinence, erectile dysfunction, damage to bladder and bowel)?*

+ *What will be the best treatment center for us?*

In the scientific literature there are differences of opinion about which treatment options offer the best cure or cancer containment rates. I spent five hours a day for a week evaluating various studies:

+ National Comprehensive Cancer Network Clinical Practice Guidelines in Oncology, Prostate Cancer, *Version 4.2011.*

+ *"Is There a Standard of Care for Pathologic Stage T3 Prostate Cancer?" by Ian M. Thompson, Catherine M. Tangen, and Eric A. Klein, published in the* Journal of Clinical Oncology, *June 20, 2009, Vol. 27, No. 18 (pp. 2898-2899).*

+ *"Preventing and Treating the Side Effects of Testosterone Deprivation Therapy in Men with Prostate Cancer: A Guide for Patients and Physicians," by Brad Guess, edited from* PCRI Insights, *November 2007, Vol. 10, No. 4.*

+ *"Radiotherapy Combined with Hormonal Therapy in Prostate Cancer: The State of the Art," by Piotr Milecki, Piotr Martenka, Andrzej Antczak, and Zbigniew Kwias, published in* Cancer Management and Research, *October 11, 2010, Vol. 2 (pp. 243-253).*

✦ *"Prostate Disorders: Your Personal Guide to Prevention, Diagnosis, and Treatment," by H. Ballentine Carter, M.D.,* The Johns Hopkins White Papers, *page 37, 2012.*

To help us in our decision making we scheduled a second-opinion consultation with the radiation oncologist at City of Hope, in hopes of finding a definitive treatment approach that we could live with.

The questions remain: How do you make the best decision for you and your loved one? How do you avoid anxiety and fear and stay in the moment?

I can tell you that it's very hard. My husband and I had a long talk during brunch today. We discussed our feelings about radiation with ADT. We are both very concerned about the potential serious side effects of two years on ADT. We do not want to take those risks, which increase over time.

I shared with my husband the recommendations about food and exercise for cancer patients that I gleaned from the three books I am reading:

✦ Life Over Cancer: The Block Center Program for Integrative Cancer Treatment, *by Keith I. Block, M.D.*

✦ Super Immunity: The Essential Nutrition Guide for Boosting Your Body's Defenses to Live Longer, Stronger, and Disease Free, *by Joel Fuhrman, M.D.*

✦ Anticancer: A New Way of Life, *by David Servan-Schreiber, M.D., Ph.D.*

My husband has a hard time reading the books. He finds them frightening and depressing. He prefers that I summarize them.

So we discussed the incorporation of foods with anti-cancer qualities and a reduction in the foods that are known to feed the growth of cancer cells and malignancy. I also told him the Block Center recommendation that he exercise for one hour a day, seven days a week.

"I won't do it! I'll get burned out. I'll get bored. I can't make myself do it....I can't hear any more about cancer. I don't want it to be the center of my life. This is all discouraging. I keep getting disappointed. I don't want to get let down again. I don't want to waste this good time in my life—when I feel fit and healthy—talking and thinking about cancer. I don't know how much time I have, and I want to enjoy it."

I told him I get overwhelmed and discouraged too. I told him I, too, have to take breaks from cancer, sometimes for days. I throw myself into gardening for four hours—just to pull weeds and feel the soil, to be quiet in nature and feel the sun. I read a good book. I go to strenuous yoga classes. I walk and play with our dog. I do a creative project. I enjoy my sessions with clients.

After our discussion we took naps and then had a really fun date of going to a new sushi restaurant and a fun mystery movie, holding hands, kissing, and laughing.

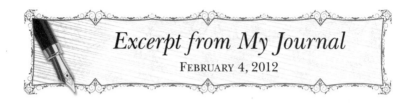

Excerpt from My Journal
FEBRUARY 4, 2012

DEAREST LORD,

The nightmare continues: My husband's second post-surgical PSA test, taken in a routine physical with his general practitioner, was **3.3! The cancer is still here and is very aggressive and fast moving. It has increased by one full PSA point in sixteen days!**

This is really, really scary news. Are we ever going to get a break in the bad news? We keep trying to hold on to HOPE—that the cancer is not as bad as we thought, that some of the dietary changes we are making will boost my husband's immune system, that the next planned treatment will give us a cure. Each time we HOPE, we are caught by surprise with more bad news.

Last week we met with the radiation oncologist and his fellow at City of Hope for a second opinion. They recommended a combination of dual blockade ADT and a seven- to seven-and-a-half-week course of radiation therapy at the highest possible dose. We decided to accept that recommendation and this facility for our treatment. We chose City of Hope for specific reasons:

+ *Unlike a community hospital that treats a variety of medical problems, City of Hope primarily specializes in treating cancer.*

+ *Every possible treatment and service is located under "one roof" on their large, beautiful campus.*

+ *The radiation oncology department treats a large number of prostate cancer patients each week. Johns Hopkins recommends getting radiation treatment at a center that treats a large number of patients with your particular diagnosis.*

+ *There is a central data department that gives physicians and patients instant access to the latest records.*

+ *All blood work and tests are done and evaluated at City of Hope, with a short turnaround.*

+ *Each physician has access to the notes and tests and recommendations of everyone else on staff.*

+ *Scheduling is handled in each department but is coordinated in a central way. Patients are handed their appointment schedule in advance.*

+ *Each physician can request a consultation with any other member of the medical staff.*

+ *Staff members in each department make personal calls to patients with reminders about appointments, changes in scheduling, etc.*

+ *City of Hope employees and volunteers greet patients and family members with a smile and a sincere desire to help.*

+ *Every detail of the grounds of the campus is meticulously cared for and planned—to give maximum comfort and spiritual/emotional support to patients and families.*

+ *Services are provided in a timely manner. There is no waiting for hours.*

On Monday we will spend the day at City of Hope, where the radiation oncologist has set up the preliminary bone scan and MRI, and where we will have our appointment to see the medical oncologist.

*It is clear that time is of the essence! Dear Lord and blessed Spirit, can't You please intervene here and **stop** or at least **slow down** the progression of the cancer until we can start the next treatment? **WE NEED DIVINE INTERVENTION!** We are your children, and we need Your help and guidance.*

I pray that we are still Stage III (T3b), that the cancer does not show up in other organs in the area of the prostate, or in distant sites, or in the bone.

*We are a unified team, and we are prepared to fight as hard or harder than it takes, but **WE NEED YOUR HELP!***

Please, please help us! You are the creator of the Universe, You have the power. Please hear our prayers and lean down to us with healing and power to beat the cancer. Please buy us time between the tests and next treatment. Please guide our deci-

sions and protect my husband from the potential serious side effects of the ADT. He is the sweetest, gentlest, most loving and sincere of men.

Please bless us. The pressure on me is beginning to take a toll. My blood work revealed a dramatic increase in my total cholesterol. Medical literature indicates there is a connection between cholesterol levels and stress. In addition, I have been getting extreme pain on the left side of my neck and the back-left side of my head. I know it is related to the long number of hours I spend reviewing the literature. The reading is intense and often frightening, but I feel I MUST do it. My husband's life is at stake!

I know that my two-times-a-week yoga class and my daily walks with Brutie are not enough to blow out the stress. I am going for a massage tomorrow and will add more cardio exercise. I MUST be grounded, healthy and strong, to support my husband in the days and months ahead. Please bless me in my endeavors, and bless my husband with healing and grace.

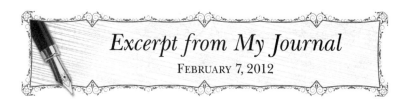

Excerpt from My Journal
FEBRUARY 7, 2012

MONDAY, **STATE OF GRACE DAY,** CITY OF HOPE:

Everything seemed to come together for our good today. We started the day with blood work. Then we had our meeting *with the medical oncologist and his fellow. We told him about the second post-surgical PSA score of 3.3, and he recommended a dual course of androgen deprivation therapy—Casodex for 21 days and Lupron for one year—combined with radiation therapy. The Casodex will prevent the "testosterone bounce" caused by the Lupron.*

The doctor said this combination would give us a 30 percent chance of cure. If we fell into the other 70 percent, my husband could be treated with intermittent androgen deprivation therapy and other choices of drugs, with the possibility of "decades and decades of living with, managing the cancer."

We decided to begin the first Lupron injection today; it will last for three months. The doctor ordered the Casodex pills to be ready at our pharmacy tonight. I asked him about getting the proper doses of calcium and Vitamin D to help prevent osteoporosis, and he said Citracal would offer the daily requirement of 1,500 mg of calcium and 800 IU of Vitamin D.

In addition, the doctor ordered a bone density test as a baseline evaluation of any osteoporosis caused by the medication. He also scheduled all the remaining Lupron injections and lab work throughout the year of therapy.

We were overjoyed and relieved to have started a definitive, aggressive attack against the cancer. The doctor's approach seemed "middle of the road" and one we could live with. It sounded so much better than two years of Lupron, with Casadex, which had been suggested by the radiation oncologist.

The doctor said the main potential side effects of the combined ADT treatment are: hot flashes, erectile dysfunction, weight gain, muscle loss, and osteoporosis. He recommended exercise at least three times a week, incorporating weights.

The rest of the day we worked the City of Hope system like a finely tuned Swiss watch. We were scheduled for a bone scan and a CT scan. We had to go back and forth from the hospital radiology department to the radiation department to the scheduling department. We moved quickly between buildings and departments and felt at home at City of Hope. We were there all day, from 8:00 a.m. to 5:00 p.m., but on the drive home we felt confident and peaceful.

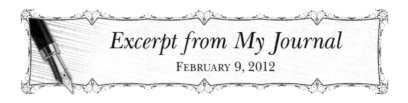

Excerpt from My Journal
FEBRUARY 9, 2012

FOR THE NEXT TWO DAYS MY HUSBAND AND I WENT ABOUT OUR daily lives with confidence and renewed enthusiasm. He was on the medications that were starving and killing the cancer. He incorporated a third day of exercise and added weight work. He was eating the anti-cancer foods and taking the Citracal.

I added another day of exercise and a dance class to my routine and had a massage, with a plan to have a massage every week.

I was proud that my husband was in warrior mode with his treatment, and I looked forward to him starting radiation on

February 21. With renewed energy and focus I was able to complete accounting tasks for my business and approve the new architectural plans for replacing the doors and windows in my minka in Santa Fe.

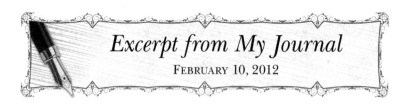

Excerpt from My Journal
FEBRUARY 10, 2012

LORD, WHERE ARE YOU? WHAT EFFECT ARE MY PRAYERS HAVING? Where is the hope? What is the use of my faith when we were, again, caught by surprise at City of Hope?

We arrived on time for our blood work, then met with our two radiation oncologists. The first one was reviewing the results of the bone and CT scans. He said, "The bone scan was negative for cancer." We were relieved and I said, "My prayers have been answered."

Then he said, "But the CT scan shows an enlarged pelvic lymph node, which means the cancer has probably spread there. Fortunately, we had already planned to radiate that area. But there is another suspicious lymph node and some spot by the lung. Have you had a cold? This machine is very sensitive and may have registered that." We weren't feeling too bad at that point.

Then the other doctor came in and things changed. He said, "The bone scan was negative, but the MRI you are having today may pick up something the bone scan did not. I recommend that we do a CT biopsy of the pelvic lymph node. If it turns out to be cancer, then we should do a higher dose of radiation to that area than we had planned."

*My husband immediately said, "**I won't have a biopsy. That is final!**" I was stunned by his response, but at the same time I knew it was important for him to take control of the decision making. He added, "No biopsy. We will move ahead with the radiation doses as planned."*

Still in a daze I asked the doctor, "If you increased the radiation to the pelvic lymph nodes, that would increase potential damage to the bladder and rectum?"

He said, "Yes."

Then I asked him, "If the MRI picks up something in the bone, how does that affect things?"

The doctor answered, "Then the staging of the cancer has to be changed to Stage IV. And that might affect the treatment plans. We should get the results by next Tuesday, and if I see something I will call you."

*My husband said to me, "**Stop asking questions. I don't want to hear this!**"*

The doctors left, and we were in another state of shock and disbelief! We sat speechless, waiting for my husband to be called for his imaging test and MRI. I was sick to my stomach, overwhelmed. I couldn't read or think another thing about cancer.

*Lord, again I ask You, **WHERE ARE YOU?** Why can't You be helping us defeat this cancer? I have prayed earnestly that we get our fair chance at the most effective treatment, which is the combination of androgen deprivation therapy and radiation therapy.*

*Please, please, please Blessed Lord, **don't let the MRI show any cancer in the BONE!** Don't deny our chance to have radiation therapy. Don't let my husband have Stage IV cancer.* ***GIVE US HOPE; GIVE US A CHANCE. WE NEED YOU!***

To help me understand the cancer staging system, I turned to the Johns Hopkins White Papers, page 37, for clarification:

(National Cancer Institute)
TNM CANCER STAGING SYSTEM —
(Tumor, Node, Metastasis)

T3: Tumor extends through the prostate capsule and may involve the seminal vesicles

T3a: Tumor extends through the capsule but does not involve the seminal vesicles

T3b: Tumor has spread to the seminal vesicles

T4: Tumor has invaded adjacent structures (other than the seminal vesicles), such as the bladder neck, rectum, or pelvic wall

N0: Cancer has not spread to any lymph nodes

N1: Cancer has spread to one or more regional lymph nodes (nodes in pelvic region)

M0: No distant metastasis

M1: *Distant metastasis*

M1a: *Cancer has spread to distant lymph nodes*

M1b: *Cancer has spread to the bones*

M1c: *Cancer has spread to other organs, with or without bone involvement*

To help me understand the difference between the words "staging" and "stages," I went to the National Cancer Institute website: www.cancer.gov/cancertopics/pdq/treatment/prostate/Patient/page 2. I found this very helpful explanation:

*The process used to find out if cancer has spread within the prostate or to other parts of the body is called **staging**. The following tests and procedures may be used in the staging process: bone scan, CT scan, MRI, pelvic lymphadenectomy, surgical pathology reports, PSA test, and Gleason scores.*

*The following **stages** are used for prostate cancer:*

Stage I: *cancer is found in the prostate only*

Stage II: *cancer is more advanced than Stage I, but has not spread outside the prostate*

Stage III: *cancer has spread beyond the outer layer of the prostate and may have spread to the seminal vesicles.*

Stage IV: *cancer has spread beyond the seminal vesicles to nearby tissue or organs, such as the rectum, bladder, or pelvic wall; or cancer may have spread to nearby lymph nodes; or cancer may have spread to distant parts of the body, which may include lymph nodes or bones.*

Taking this information and analyzing my husband's surgical pathology results, he is currently a Stage III prostate cancer patient, as he has T3b, N0, M0 in the TNM Cancer Staging System. We don't yet know if there is metastasis to the lymph nodes or the bones. The bone scan and CT scan were negative, but we must wait for the MRI results to know if he will maintain his Stage III status.

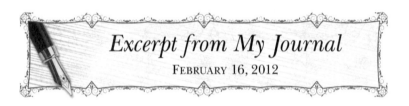

Excerpt from My Journal
FEBRUARY 16, 2012

OVER THIRTY YEARS AGO, WHEN I WAS AN ONCOLOGY SOCIAL worker, I wrote that the families of cancer patients are at high risk for developing cancer themselves.

Today I got a call from my primary care physician stating: "I just got your Pap test results back. There isn't any sign of cancer, but you tested positive for HPV. Don't worry, you don't have cancer. But your HPV shows some irregular cells that, left untreated, could become cancer of the cervix. I am referring you to a gynecologist in our group, who will use a scope to examine your cervix and remove or cauterize any damage the HPV may have caused."

I was stunned! Another medical scare, and this time it is ME!

Dealing with my husband's cancer is the most stressful event in my adult life. *Fear and powerlessness have been* *with me nearly every day since his diagnosis on 11-11-11. Three solid, unrelenting months.*

FEAR AND POWERLESSNESS ARE DEBILITATING!

I have tried to use all my holistic self-care skills to cope. I have journaled, prayed, done yoga and exercise, gardened. But the stress has been more than I can manage. Please lead me, dear Spirit, into other ways I can restore my health and inner balance. One good idea is for me to call my former therapist and schedule some sessions. Yes, even therapists need their own therapist.

I thank You, Lord, that we did not get a phone call from City of Hope about any surprises from my husband's MRI. That has to mean that no cancer was found in his bones, and therefore there is no reason why he can't begin his radiation as planned on 2-21-12.

This is wonderful! We are no longer helpless. We have treatment options that can help us kill the cancer, and we can resume the normal flow of our lives. I know this will eliminate the daily fear I have been carrying and help my body heal.

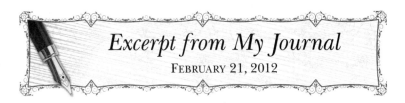

Excerpt from My Journal
FEBRUARY 21, 2012

DRIVING WITH MY HUSBAND TO HIS FIRST RADIATION TREATMENT, I told him: "I am ready to pass the baton to you. I shepherded you through the first three months of your treatment, going with you to every appointment, doing research, helping you recover from surgery. Now it is time for you to take over."

He told me he was ready: "I can go to the radiation treatments by myself. It's something that I will organize into a routine. I will work out in the early morning, drive to my treatments, then come home, rest, and attend to my business. I am looking forward to it. It is something I will do for myself. Five times a week for eight weeks. That's the schedule. In addition, I plan to take private classical guitar lessons. Playing the guitar is something I love, and I know it will be good for me. And, yes, I am praying to God nearly every day."

When we arrived for my husband's first treatment, he told the radiation oncologist: "I do not want to radiate the pelvic lymph nodes at a higher dose than had been originally planned. I do not want to risk damage to the nearby bladder and rectum."

We had been given a brochure and a DVD that explained the radiation treatment and possible side effects. At this point my husband had regained his bladder control nearly 100 percent, and he was eager to preserve it.

My husband was called for his treatment, and it was finished in a matter of minutes. What a relief! I think it's pretty neat that City of Hope gives each patient receiving radiation therapy a picture ID, which must be verified, before they receive each treatment. This is in addition to wearing their wristband

and having to state their birth date. Every precaution is taken to ensure that the right patient receives the right treatment.

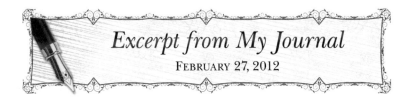

Excerpt from My Journal
FEBRUARY 27, 2012

DEAREST LORD,

Nervous though I was, I went to my appointment at the gynecologist. The attending nurse told me that they were probably not going to perform the colposcopy, as the Pap test was normal and only showed the presence of HPV. They thought, since I had never had an abnormal Pap smear in my entire life, I could wait six months and then have another one.

I told the doctor I would prefer to have the colposcopy today, as I was worried about the irregular cells that had been identified.

She explained to me that I have probably had HPV in my system for years, in a dormant state, but that some great stress in my life could have activated it.

Just as I suspected! I told her about my husband's diagnosis of prostate cancer three months ago, and she agreed that the stress had activated the HPV.

The caring manner of this woman doctor was exactly what I needed. She understood the strain of my husband's cancer and was very gentle and reassuring with me. Her behavior was very different than that of my internist, who did not even blink when I told him about my husband's cancer. He didn't ask me one single question or offer me any consolation.

The doctor performed the colposcopy and said she would have the results in a week.

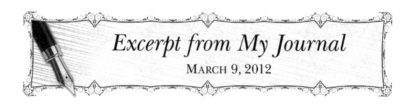

Excerpt from My Journal
MARCH 9, 2012

Yesterday was a "state of grace" day for me, Lord. The results of my second Pap test were negative. There is no cancer in my body. I was, however, given a second diagnosis of Lichen Sclerosus, an autoimmune disorder. I believe it, too, was a reaction to the stress of my husband's cancer.

In my second session with my therapist, she was amazed how much I had changed in one week. In the first session, strain was evident throughout my body. After that session I did some reading in Women's Bodies, Women's Wisdom: Creating Physical and Emotional Health and Healing, *by Christiane Northrup, M.D., and was encouraged by her theory that women's gynecological problems are often related to stress, feelings of being powerless or victimized, and trauma experienced at various phases of their sexual development.*

At Women to Women health care center—which Northrup co-founded with Marcelle Pick, OB/GYN, NP, in the 1980s—great changes and elimination of problems occur when women are able to connect their emotions to their bodies and adopt forgiveness, self-love, and self-empowerment into their lifestyles. Northrup also recommends a high-potency multivitamin and mineral supplement.

During my energy movement session with my therapist today (which incorporated deep breathing, deep exhalation, and total body relaxation), she said that energy was flowing beautifully throughout my body, and that I looked radiant and fully alive. She told me I had achieved that change within myself even though nothing in my outer environment had changed. She told me to remember that, and to recreate it within myself whenever I need it.

When I got home I was so relaxed that I invented some new recipes:

Quesadilla: *Sliced banana, sliced avocado, shredded cheese, tortilla, sunflower seeds. Spray olive oil on tortilla, add mixture, heat on grill. Delicious!*

Stir Fry: *1 cup of quinoa (red and yellow) that has been rinsed, drained, and boiled 20 minutes in 2 cups of water; Brussels sprouts that have been cleaned and quartered; 1 cup of sliced mushrooms; 1 bunch of purple kale that has been rinsed and diced, with the large veins removed; 2 tablespoons olive oil; half-cup of water. Heat 3-5 minutes in covered skillet, top with cheese. Heat until melted. Serve and enjoy!*

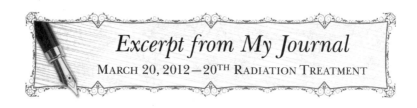

Excerpt from My Journal
MARCH 20, 2012—20TH RADIATION TREATMENT

WE HAVE SETTLED INTO THE SAFE COCOON OF CITY OF HOPE for this phase of our treatment. The pressure is off in terms of the need to do research, evaluate facilities, interview doctors, or learn about equipment and protocols.

As this facility's name implies, we have hope and feel safe. Now we can go back to living our lives like normal people, without the word "cancer" in our everyday vocabulary.

There is a relief from fear, and we are finding joy once again on many levels and in many ways. I can say that I have never loved my husband as much as during this experience with cancer. Each day, each moment, each activity has been heightened with appreciation and love.

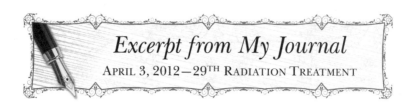

Excerpt from My Journal
APRIL 3, 2012—29TH RADIATION TREATMENT

MY HUSBAND DECIDED, BECAUSE OF THE ENLARGED PELVIC lymph node that was detected by the MRI, to increase the number of targeted doses to that area by nine more sessions. He wanted to make sure to use the radiation to full advan-

tage—to give him the best chance of killing all the cancer. His radiation oncologists and his medical oncologists agreed.

Throughout his treatments he has had very few side effects from the radiation: occasional diarrhea, some urinary leakage, and a small pain pinpointed on his right lower abdomen. He has experienced some fatigue but has always continued to do his full schedule of work, exercise, and family activities.

I have been very impressed with his strong spirit and heart, and am very proud of him.

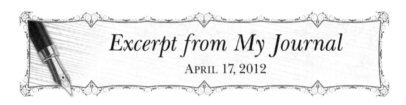

Excerpt from My Journal
APRIL 17, 2012

MY HUSBAND COMPLETED HIS LAST RADIATION TREATMENT today. The radiation department staff took a picture of him inside and standing beside the radiation machine, then gave him a gold Medal of Honor. He was very proud.

I admire my husband and love him with all my heart. Throughout his radiation treatments he worked out at the gym doing weight and cardio training, maintaining a solid, eye-catching physique and stamina. He worked full time in his company and had a positive, powerful attitude and behavior.

*In his last visit with his radiation oncologist, the doctor said: "You are doing fantastic. Your post-radiation PSA result was **less than 0.04 - undetectable level of cancer.** Your testos-*

terone level is 40.9. You are in great hands with your medical oncologist, and he will take care of anything else if need be."

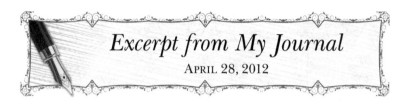

Excerpt from My Journal
APRIL 28, 2012

THE DAYS OF APRIL HAVE BEEN VERY GOOD TO US. WE HAVE *not really been thinking about the cancer. My husband has driven himself to the daily radiation treatments, and I have been free to prepare the soil and plant four vegetable gardens, stain the perimeter fences around the yard, and stain my two Japanese tea houses.*

I would say that gardening is one of the most powerful spiritual and mental activities I can do. No matter if I am depressed, when I work in my garden—touch the soil; pull weeds; plant vegetables, flowers, and trees; and work hard physically with my shovel, rake, and wheelbarrow—I become stronger physically, mentally, emotionally, and spiritually, and I am blessed by the beauty I create.

I have felt healthy, happy, peaceful, and optimistic this month. I made a trip to Santa Fe to survey the successful completion of the new windows and doors in my minka—which was enormously satisfying. Likewise, my husband has engaged in activities that nourish him: classical guitar lessons and daily practice, reading adventure books that capture his imagination, doing his exercise regime.

*Along-the-Journey
Recommendations for the Prostate
Cancer Patient and His Loved Ones*

BY THIS PHASE IN OUR JOURNEY MY HUSBAND AND I had lived through a variety of treatments for five months. It was a long period of time, filled with ups and downs, hope and disappointments—and enduring it required a lot of fortitude. For that reason I am going to devote this set of recommendations to a section I call "Develop the Characteristics of a Warrior."

Many prostate cancer patients will have shorter periods of treatment, and perhaps only one form of treatment. It will depend on the severity of the prostate cancer and the associated Gleason scores. Lower Gleason scores may warrant only "active surveillance." Medium-range Gleason scores may indicate either surgery or radiation alone. For those with the highest Gleason scores, like my husband, a variety of treatments will be necessary.

Regardless of the length and type of treatment(s), I do believe that when battling cancer, both the patient and his loved ones must be armed with character qualities that can carry them through the process to victory. Both patient and loved one(s) need to become *warriors*.

Develop the Characteristics of a Warrior

Stamina

Winning the battle against cancer is not for the faint of heart. You must develop the heart, spirit, and stamina of a warrior. Whatever your personality style, when you first hear the diagnosis of cancer your whole system goes into shock. The word "cancer" alone is enough to blow you over, knock you down, take your breath away.

Shortly after learning the diagnosis you must pick yourself up and dust yourself off. Dr. Keith I. Block, in his book *Life Over Cancer*, states that dealing with cancer is like preparing for a marathon.

Cancer is an unknown variable. The doctors don't know from minute to minute what it will do. Sometimes the treatments are brief, sometimes they are extended. Sometimes there are few side effects of the treatment, sometimes there are many.

As you and your family live with cancer, you must develop **stamina** in your body, mind, emotions, and spirit. If you are strong in all of these respects, you will boost the functioning of your immune system and increase the odds of a positive outcome.

Hope

In your battle against cancer you are going to need a boatload of hope. The definition of hope: "desire accompanied by expectation of or belief in fulfillment."

I cannot stress enough the importance of **hope**. It is an expectation of good that originates in your mind, then trickles down to your heart, your emotions, your body, and your spirit. It sets up a positive expectation that can become a self-fulfilling prophecy.

With hope we can relax in the moment, trust the treatment plan, recover from disappointment, move on to the next treatment, catch our breath, and rejoice in each day. With hope we can return our attention to our families, our jobs, our children and grandchildren, our pets, our friends, our community. With hope we can let go of fear and concentrate on matters at hand. With hope we can sleep peacefully at night and relax in our bodies.

DO NOT LET ANYONE TAKE AWAY YOUR HOPE. Sometimes doctors will be very pessimistic. Sometimes family members will give up. Particularly if you're the patient, you must hold onto your hope of cure or hope that your cancer can be managed for years to come. If you lose your hope, you lose your heart, your stamina, your will to live. Your body will follow.

Faith

At the very least a warrior must have faith in himself, his armor, and his weapons. To be successful in battle he must believe he can defeat the enemy.

The definition of **faith** is: "believing in that which you cannot yet see." On a very deep level you must have faith in the body's ability to heal itself. For this reason I encourage you to read the books I have referenced previously that discuss the design and functioning of the immune system.

You must also have faith in the treatments at the time they are being received. Suspend your fear, suspend your doubts, and have faith that they will help kill the cancer.

Then there's the area of faith that there is a Higher Power who can assist you in your battle with cancer. It is said that "there are no atheists in a fox hole." Whatever your personal belief system prior to the cancer diagnosis, I highly recommend that you explore the matter of faith once the diagnosis has been made. Cancer is an enemy, and you are in a fox hole of sorts.

Maybe it's a good time to suspend your doubt or disbelief, call out to God or Higher Power (however you would define Him, Her, It), and ask for some help.

What I'm talking about doesn't involve belonging to any church or following any particular religion. It's as simple as listening to your heart, your needs, in the battle you are fighting with cancer and asking Higher Power to help you.

Personally, I don't know how my husband and I could have gotten this far, this successfully, if it had not been for the help we received from God. No matter how discouraging things got on a given day, with a given medical report or test result, we were always given a sense of inner peace, a release from our anxiety, and the ability to trust in the moment.

Assertiveness

A warrior cannot be timid. He must know his mind and be able to speak it. He must be able to assess alternatives and make a choice. He cannot be intimidated by the fear of what other people will think. He must be decisive.

At this point in his treatment my husband made a decision that went against his doctor's recommendation. The radiation oncologist wanted to biopsy the suspicious pelvic lymph node. My husband adamantly refused. He simply did not want another surgical procedure. The doctor went along with his decision.

My husband was, however, willing to have the MRI, which might have revealed that the cancer had spread to the bone. We were blessed when the results showed no metastasis to the bone, which maintained his T3b status and allowed him to be treated with dual blockade ADT and radiation. The protocol for Stage IV is that the patient be treated with androgen deprivation therapy alone, no salvage radiation.

When my husband finished his radiation his PSA level was "undetectable." Would he have had the same result with only ADT? We will never know.

I encourage patients and family members to carefully evaluate all the treatment options and then make your best decision. Listen to all the medical advice. Read as much of the medical literature as you can tolerate. Pray for good judgment and guidance. But in the end it is *your* decision, *your* life. Don't be afraid of making the doctors angry if you disagree with them.

Good Self-Care Skills

A professional warrior knows that **he must be disciplined in the care of his body and his mind.** Good armor and weapons alone will not win a battle. The warrior's body must be strong and healthy. It must be well fed and rested.

For the prostate cancer patient I recommend the following self-care skills:

+ Take responsibility for the kind of food you put into your body. Don't rely on your family members to monitor what you eat. Read the books I have recommended that discuss anti-cancer foods, and try to incorporate them into your diet. By the same token, try to reduce your intake of foods that promote cancer growth. Eat in moderation.

+ Devise some kind of regular exercise schedule and routine that will produce cardio stamina, strength, and muscle tone as well as weight management. Exercise will reduce tension and enhance your moods by giving you endorphins. It will also give you more self-confidence in your battle with cancer. If your body is strong, your mind and spirit will be too.

+ Take time to rest when your body tells you it is tired. Rest is recuperative for your immune system, and it often elevates your mood.

+ Engage in activities that promote peacefulness, mental challenge, stress reduction, creativity, and joy.

+ Explore ways to strengthen your spirit. Find books that inspire you, help other people, meditate, pray, write, spend time in nature and with pets if you have them, do creative projects, spend quiet time with your Self. Develop "eyes that can see and ears that can hear" the wonders of spirit. The ways of the spirit must be seen and heard by your *heart*, not by your *mind*. To access your heart you must spend quiet time with your Self and turn inward. In the quiet, listen for messages from God, your spirit, your intuition.

+ When you are struggling with your emotions or scary thoughts about cancer, talk to someone you trust (your wife/partner/family member/friend/support group members/therapist). When you talk, you release tension from your body and your heart; you receive love, encouragement, and insight; your stamina, courage, and hope return. Allowing yourself to cry is another way to release frustration, anger, disappointment, and hurt. Crying does not make you less of a man. On the contrary, it shows that you are strong enough to admit that you are vulnerable. And vulnerability is an

essential ingredient in being able to love yourself and other people.

+ Give love, hugs, and appreciation to the people
in your life. The more you give, the more you
will receive.

+ Remind yourself that **you are a warrior** and
that you will fight the cancer with all your
might. Be positive, hopeful, and courageous.

+ Set some personal goals for yourself that extend
beyond your cancer treatment. Think of things
that will challenge, excite, and inspire you. These
goals will create forward momentum and energy
that will stimulate health in your body, mind,
emotions, and spirit. Be specific with your
goals: What are they? How will you feel when
you achieve them? What new ones will you set?
Use these goals as part of your positive visualizations. Spend time thinking about them.
**Having a vision for your future will aid in
surviving cancer.**

For the prostate cancer patient's loved ones I recommend the following self-care skills:

You, like me, are in the position of supporting your
man in the battle with prostate cancer. We know

that it is a long, hard, exhausting journey filled with a roller coaster of emotions and huge physical demands. As such, over time your own body will become vulnerable to developing medical problems. The stress of the cancer will localize in any part of your body that has a predisposition to problems: your heart, your lungs, your back, your intestines, or your immune system, to name a few possibilities.

IF YOU DO NOT TAKE CARE OF YOUR OWN BODY, you too can develop cancer or some other form of life-threatening illness. **IF YOU DO NOT TAKE CARE OF YOUR EMOTIONS**, you can fall into a depression or suffer from anxiety. **IF YOU DO NOT FIND A WAY TO MAINTAIN BALANCE** in your life, you will develop burnout.

You must find ways to take as good care of yourself as you do of your patient. A few ideas:

+ Establish a support system of people who can help you with the added demands in your life.

+ Exercise for a half-hour a day, three times a week.

+ Make some quiet time for yourself when you can recharge. A hot bath, fun magazines, coffee or lunch with a friend, time in nature, a nap,

fun movies, a manicure/pedicure or a massage—all of these activities can fit the bill.

+ Go for regular medical checkups.

+ If you are too tired to make healthy meals, buy
some and bring them home.

+ Take breaks from thinking about the cancer.
Engage your mind in reading books or meditations that nourish your spirit. Lose yourself
in activities that make you feel peaceful and
happy. Take vacations.

+ Consider getting a therapist, or use a journal
to release your emotions and maintain your
relationship with your Self.

+ Find some ways to strengthen your spirit: prayer,
yoga, meditation. Even paying attention to the
messages in your dreams is spiritual support.

+ Hugging your husband, your kids, your grandchildren, your friends, or your pets releases oxytocin
into your bloodstream. Oxytocin gives you a sense
of well-being and relaxation and reduces your heart
rate—much like endorphins do.

+ Crying is another way to release stress, frustration, disappointment, and fatigue. It is not a

sign of weakness. Allowing the tears to stream down your cheeks is like a cloud burst that releases energy and nourishes the earth. Afterwards, there is a sense of peace and quiet.

Flexibility

Any commander of warriors must be prepared to rethink, retreat, or regroup when the initial battle plan is unsuccessful. He cannot be attached to only one strategy. When presented with a small defeat he must take time to design a new plan of action. He is not worried that losing a minor battle will cost him the war. He and his officers will weigh the options, look for weaknesses in the enemy, avail themselves of new weaponry, design new battle plans.

The warrior must consider recommendations from his chiefs of staff. He needs to be humble and accept the fact that he may have to do something he never thought he would do. He must remember the warning, "Never underestimate the power of your opponent."

Cancer is a slippery, strong opponent. Just when you think you have it cornered it finds an escape route and pops up somewhere else. A treatment that seemed pretty sure of killing it can prove to be unsuccessful. This does not mean you will lose the war.

You must not be disheartened if the first treatment plan is unsuccessful in killing all the cancer. Take a deep breath, cry if you feel like it, acknowledge your disappointment, then move forward. **Fighting cancer takes courage and flexibility.** Reconsider ideas that you originally rejected. Don't be stubborn. Don't be stuck in your own ego. Be humble and take time to reconsider every option. It's fine to change your mind.

Initially my husband rejected the idea of surgery. His heart was set on killing the cancer with radiation. When he finally understood that his cancer was too dangerous and too aggressive, he changed his mind and went with the robotic-assisted radical prostatectomy as his first treatment.

When the radiation oncologist suggested extra targeted radiation to the suspicious pelvic lymph node, my husband originally said no. When he finally understood that he would be missing an opportunity to kill cancer that might have spread to that area, he changed his mind and requested the extra radiation. Each of these decisions may have saved his life.

My husband also initially fought my recommendations to change our diet and increase his exercise.

The fact that he ultimately made these changes may well have contributed to his current progress.

If your initial, traditional treatments of surgery, radiation, and androgen deprivation therapy do not kill all the cancer, be open to participating in clinical trials and trying new approaches recommended by your treatment team.

You might also explore alternative therapies that will complement your medical treatment, but I don't recommend that you stop the medical treatments. One adjunct treatment is acupuncture. Others are diet, psychotherapy, and meditation.

Determination

The warriors who are **determined to live**—against all odds and punishment/challenges from nature, man, and the inner self—are the mostly likely to survive. In fighting the battle with your cancer, you must be absolutely certain about your resolve to survive. No matter how many times you are knocked down, you must get up again. When you feel like quitting, you must push through. No matter how bad or discouraged you are from the treatments or test results, you must hold onto your determination to live. It is a matter of committing your mind and spirit to the task of survival. Following that commitment, you must be resourceful in your actions: "What can I do to increase my chances of survival? What areas of my life do I need to change?" Never underestimate the power of your mind and your spirit!

If all your efforts and treatments are unsuccessful in the end, you will be at peace within yourself, knowing you fought as gallantly as possible and have the right to finally let go. At the Cancer Counseling and Research Center in Ft. Worth, Texas, the Simontons' research showed that the Stage IV cancer patients who were most determined and most independent lived longer, with less pain and higher quality of life. None of us knows if we will eventually lose the battle with cancer or some other disease. We are all going to die of something, at some time. Your determination to live, however, and the actions you take to support that determination will strongly influence the quality of your life and the transition to the next life.

Examples of Inspirational Real-Life Warriors

Four inspirational nonfiction books that my husband read to me on the weekends embody all the characteristics of the warrior. These books are true-life accounts of courageous warriors.

Two of the books are about Sir Ernest Shackleton, an Irish Antarctic explorer, and his mission to save his men who were stranded on Elephant Island in 1914 when their ship the *Endurance* was trapped in the ice and destroyed. Another book is about American Army Air Corps members and National Guardsmen trapped in Greenland in 1942 when their airplanes went down, and the valiant efforts to save them. The fourth book is about the amazing 1936 Olympic marathon runner and Army Air Corps bombardier Louis Zamperini, an American who survived forty-seven days in a lifeboat when his B-24 was shot down in the Pacific during World War II, and two years of torture in a Japanese POW camp.

Endurance: Shackleton's Incredible Voyage, by Alfred Lansing

The Endurance: Shackleton's Legendary Antarctic Expedition, by Caroline Alexander

Frozen in Time: An Epic Story of Survival and a Modern Quest for Lost Heroes of World War II, by Mitchell Zuckoff

Unbroken: A World War II Story of Survival, Resilience, and Redemption, by Laura Hillenbrand

I highly recommend these books for men and families battling prostate cancer. All of the men featured in the books were faced with impossible odds of survival and had to draw on every fiber of their beings for the strength, endurance, and imagination required to survive. Moreover, each of these men prayed for God to assist him.

I conclude this chapter with a quote from *Unbroken* (page 148) in which the author analyzes Louie and his two raft mates, all of whom are lost on the sea:

"Though all three men faced the same hardship, their differing perceptions of it appeared to be shaping their fates. Louie and Phil's hope displaced their fear and inspired them to work toward their survival, and each success renewed their physical and emotional vigor. Mac's resignation seemed to paralyze him, and the less he participated in their efforts to survive, the more he slipped. Though he did the least, as the days passed, it was he who faded the most. Louie and Phil's optimism, and Mac's hopelessness, were becoming self-fulfilling."

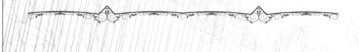

CHAPTER SEVEN

Androgen Deprivation Therapy and Beyond

THIS CHAPTER COVERS NINE MONTHS OF ANDROGEN DEP-rivation therapy post-radiation, as well as time beyond. The story is continuing to unfold. I am sure we have more lessons to learn, and perhaps we will face some more challenges too.

What we have learned so far is that God is with us; we are still One Body, Four Legs with the spirit of a warrior; we have a wonderful treatment team at City of Hope; and that life must be celebrated in the moment. We do not know what the future holds for us, but we hold on to our **hope** and determination to fight the cancer.

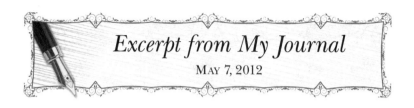

Excerpt from My Journal
MAY 7, 2012

MY HUSBAND'S SECOND POST-RADIATION PSA TEST REVEALED another **"less than 0.04 – undetectable level of cancer."** *His testosterone level was 34.2. Praise God!*

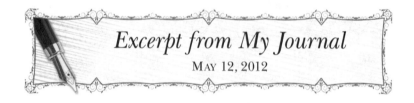

Excerpt from My Journal
MAY 12, 2012

TODAY I BEGIN WRITING THE BOOK. THESE ARE MY INITIAL *thoughts:*

"The purpose of this book is to educate, inspire, and give power to your fight against prostate cancer. It is written for the brave men who have prostate cancer and for the people who love and care for them.

This book addresses the psychological and emotional impact that prostate cancer has on the lives of those it touches.

Join one family's journey and celebrate this view of God in action."

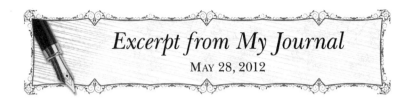

Excerpt from My Journal
MAY 28, 2012

TODAY I GOT A NOTICE FROM THE STATE OF CALIFORNIA THAT *my current property taxes are delinquent. "What? How could that happen? I'm the kind of person who always pays my bills a month ahead!"*

I went to my desk and pulled out my paperwork. Sure enough I had forgotten to pay the property taxes on my house in April. It hadn't even come to my mind. If I hadn't gotten this notice I would have forgotten them altogether.

"Where was my mind in April? How did I forget?" I realized then that I had been preoccupied with my husband's radiation treatments, the final visit with the radiation oncologist, and check-in with the medical oncologist. We had been worried about what the PSA test would reveal. Would there be any signs of cancer? Was the combination of radiation and hormone therapy successful?

"Since I forgot the California property taxes I must have forgotten the New Mexico property taxes as well." Sure enough, they had not been paid either.

This was a humbling reminder that living with cancer can wreak havoc with your ordinary life and functioning. I had to be gentle with myself and cut myself some slack.

"Don't judge yourself harshly. I know you are an organized person who likes to be in control and do things well. But you've had a lot on your mind. You've been under a tremendous strain."

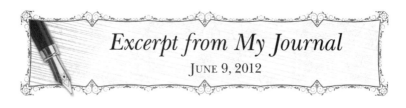

Excerpt from My Journal
JUNE 9, 2012

THE PRESSURE AND STRAIN FROM THE CANCER ARE ALWAYS HERE. As we approach the third PSA test in July I can feel the pressure mounting.

The last two months have been relatively peaceful—a period of grace when we haven't had to think about cancer because of the undetectable PSA test at the end of radiation and the one a month later. Each of us needed that break. We got back into our regular lives and had time to devote ourselves to work, exercise, family, and our individual selves.

Because the need to support my husband had diminished, I had more energy and could notice the things around me that I had neglected: the backyard fence and tea houses, which needed to be stained, as well as my body.

With each brush stroke of the stain I saw the teahouses and fences being transformed from dull and lifeless to rich and beautiful. It was as if I was transforming myself. The cancer had taken a lot out of me, and I felt dull and lifeless. The work was tedious and demanding but immensely satisfying. Another bonus with staining work is that you must stay focused in the moment or you will make a mess. I seized the opportunity to use this as a mindfulness practice: focus, breathe, notice your body, pay attention to every detail, stay in the moment, breathe.

In terms of my body, I noticed in yoga that my strength had diminished and that my arms, back, and waist muscles had begun to sag. "How did this happen? When did this happen? This won't do at all. I want my body back. I want my strength back!"

I knew that my body would recover its strength and muscles as I returned to doing strong physical labor and gardening. There's nothing I love more than working with my shovel, wheelbarrow, clippers, and paint brushes to maintain a beautiful yard and structures. These jobs give me an opportunity to control my environment even if I cannot control the cancer. I create beauty in nature and my spirit is replenished.

My husband has also benefited from this respite from cancer and treatments. During the months of radiation, four hours of each day were consumed by his commute to City of Hope and the treatment. Then he had to struggle against the fatigue and push himself to work six hours on his business, plus work out at the gym. He, too, had very little time for himself.

In the two months since he completed radiation he has felt like he is on vacation. He has four extra hours each day that are "free." I have encouraged him to use the time to relax and replenish his strength and spirit. He relishes his guitar lessons and practice, and he has become an avid nonfiction reader. I think the stories he is drawn to nourish his warrior spirit.

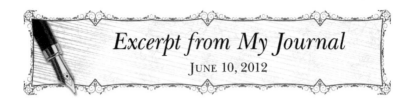

Excerpt from My Journal
June 10, 2012

WONDERFUL NEWS: ***MY HUSBAND'S CONTINENCE,*** *WHICH WAS lost halfway through his radiation treatments,* ***is returning!*** *Yesterday was the first day he did not have to change a pad!*

This is a physical and emotional breakthrough, and the return of hope and restoration. There is no reason why his continence cannot be fully restored.

Praise God! This was a true desire of his heart. He is returning to the man he was prior to the diagnosis and treatment of cancer. The temporary incontinence he has experienced the last two months must have been related to the radiation. He had faith in his bladder and urethra, and they seem to be healing.

His medical oncologist told him:

> *"Within another three months the incontinence should fully recover, especially because you recovered it after the radical prostatectomy. In terms of the pain in your right side, it is probably connected to the right lymph node that shrank during the targeted radiation treatments. Your erectile functioning may return when we complete the Lupron treatments and your testosterone returns."*

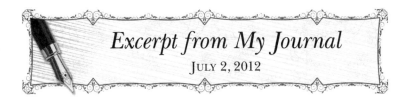

Excerpt from My Journal
JULY 2, 2012

THANKS TO THE ANTI-CANCER DIET, MY EFFORTS TO TAKE CARE of myself, my husband's apparent health, the fun things we have been doing, and the reduction of stress, my cholesterol has returned to its normal level.

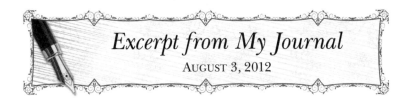

Excerpt from My Journal
AUGUST 3, 2012

MY DOG BRUTIE AND I ARE IN NEW MEXICO FOR OUR YEARLY five-week vacation. My husband will spend two and a half weeks with us and we will all drive home together. Time to rest, read all day long, take long walks in the arroyos, sleep outdoors in our minka, enjoy the beautiful sky and nature, have fun adventures, and decompress.

*My husband just phoned me with the results of his third PSA test post-radiation: **"less than 0.04 - undetectable for cancer"**! His testosterone was 25.8. His new radiation oncologist told him: "You look to be in great health! You are doing everything right. Your incontinence is better. Have another PSA test in three months, and see me again in six months."*

My husband really likes this new radiation oncologist, who took over his case when the other doctor moved out of state: "His manner gives you a warm feeling. He is quick to talk about the positive things. He came into the office with the PSA test results in his hand, smiling, and said, 'You're probably waiting to see this.' He had taken it upon himself to make me a copy."

My husband went on to say:

> *"City of Hope is a neat place to be. They are very organized and efficient. You never have to wait long. They phone ahead and remind you of your appointment. I have never been at a hospital where it is so pleasant. Every person is smiling and cheerful and can't do enough to help you. They are all on the same team with the same standard of performance. I am blessed. Coming to this place was not luck; it had to be a blessed event."*

This was the key PSA test—three months after radiation. The first two were good, but this one shows the trend. I said a prayer last night and will check back in today to give thanks.

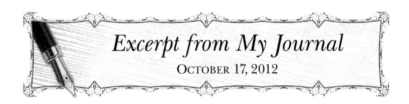

Excerpt from My Journal
OCTOBER 17, 2012

PRAISE GOD! **MY PAP TEST AND HPV TEST TAKEN TWO WEEKS ago came back normal!** *The doctor said, "Your immune system is back to normal and has cleared the HPV from your body."*

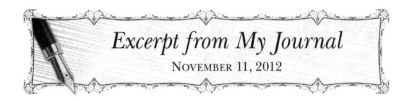

Excerpt from My Journal
NOVEMBER 11, 2012

*WHAT A WONDERFUL DAY. EXACTLY ONE YEAR AGO MY HUSBAND was diagnosed with a very aggressive, very dangerous strain of prostate cancer. Today his medical oncologist told him that his fourth PSA test was, once again, **"less than 0.04 - UNDE-TECTABLE FOR CANCER"**! His testosterone was 27.1.*

The doctor went on to say: "This is your last Lupron shot— for a total of four over the course of one year. We do not want to take a chance with going any longer as the testosterone might become permanently suppressed. There could also be other bad side effects. The real test for the cancer will be whether it returns when the testosterone climbs."

We put our trust in You, God, and vow to stay "in present time." We will bask in our good present and the fact that You have carried us through the full year since diagnosis on 11-11-11.

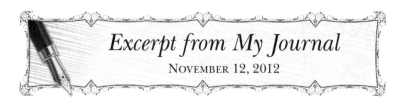

Excerpt from My Journal
November 12, 2012

Dearest Lord,

At last I am quiet and writing to You. I am exhausted, worn out, fragile, and weak. I did not notice until now that I have the classic symptoms of burnout:

- *Reactivity*
- *Irritability*
- *Fatigue*
- *Easily overwhelmed*
- *Agitation*
- *Nervousness*
- *Physical symptoms*
- *Weakness of body, mind, emotions, and spirit*

When I prayed for a scripture to guide me I was given Zechariah 4,6:

> *"Not by might, nor by power, but by My Spirit, says the Lord of Hosts—you will succeed because of My Spirit."*

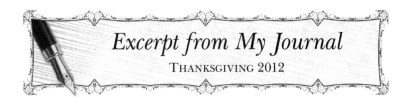

Excerpt from My Journal
THANKSGIVING 2012

I AM NOT HAPPY, LORD. I AM EXHAUSTED—BEYOND MEASURE. I am feeling no joy, no excitement, no contentment. Everything is effortful.

I knew I was too tired to prepare the big Thanksgiving meal. I pushed myself to do it for my husband—because he wanted it and was pushing me to do it. I wanted to do it for him because I love him and because he had survived a year with cancer, but I should not have done so.

Preparing and serving the meal took eight hours. Was it worth it? I really don't know. I feel half alive, half present, empty. Everything that is good has run out of me—my wit, my creativity, my laughter, my joy, my enthusiasm.

I am empty and worn out. I want to be alone so I can rest and mend and find my way back to my Self.

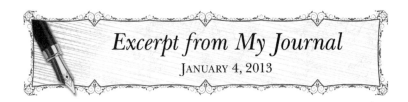

Excerpt from My Journal
JANUARY 4, 2013

THE MONTH OF DECEMBER WAS A BLUR. MY EXHAUSTION DID not abate; it only got worse. I tried to cut down on the energy

*I expended, but some things just had to be done: holiday prepa-
rations and celebrations, travel to New Mexico.*

*I continued to feel irritable and out of sorts and just wanted to
be alone—away from any demands on my dwindling strength.*

*My husband, who has been the center of my life this last year
with his cancer, became increasingly irritated and angry with
my withdrawal. He kept pushing me for MORE, which made
me only more resentful and fatigued.*

*I nearly cancelled our holiday trip to New Mexico but decided
to go at the last minute. I guess it is no surprise that I developed
a severe upper respiratory infection, which lasted a month.*

*I was totally worn out. I could not talk. Immense amounts of
dead cells filled my head and sinuses, my throat, my chest. All
I could do was blow my nose, cough, sleep. I had no appetite.*

*I said to my body: "Okay. I will give you and my spirit all the
rest you need. Go ahead and be weak. Let down, let go. I give
you permission to rest. I embrace the rest."*

*The only highlight of this experience was that my husband
really stepped up to the plate when I was sick. Each morning
he made me a hot pot of coffee and a fruit bowl, which he
served me in bed. He also started the tradition, which continues today, of reading to me and my dog the adventures of
famous explorers and rescue missions. This has become my
absolutely favorite tradition that we have on the weekends.*

In addition, he made all the meals and took me for special Christmas and New Year's dinners. He took really, really good care of me and was very patient with my long illness.

Today I am nearly well. I feel better. My joy and energy are returning. I will keep careful watch over all my needs and set limits and boundaries with demands for my time.

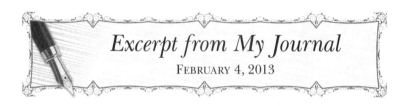

Excerpt from My Journal
FEBRUARY 4, 2013

FIFTH POST-RADIATION PSA: "LESS THAN 0.04 - UNDETECTABLE for cancer"! My husband's testosterone was 29.6.

In our meeting with the medical oncologist we asked about certain problems my husband was having: weight gain; increase in abdominal girth; and severe pain, aching, and cysts in his hands near the thumb joints. The doctor said these were probably all side effects of the Lupron and should diminish over time once my husband finishes the treatment.

We asked if my husband should have another bone scan and the doctor said, "It would not be helpful right now. We will do it in another six months."

At the end of our meeting the doctor said, "When testosterone returns, that is the crucial time to watch the PSA. We will do the sixth PSA test in three months."

Meanwhile, my husband has gone to a hand specialist, who injects Cortizone into his painful thumb joints. This gives him some relief.

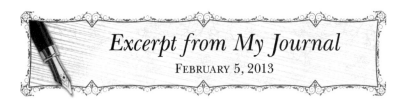

Excerpt from My Journal
FEBRUARY 5, 2013

CONCERNED WITH THE INCREASE IN THE SIZE OF HIS ABDOMEN due to the Lupron, my husband purchased the book Wheat Belly: Lose the Wheat, Lose the Weight, and Find Your Path Back to Health, *by William Davis, M.D. He will begin a gluten-free diet. In addition, he has modified his workouts to target this area.*

I have to say that I admire my husband's warrior spirit and the way he takes responsibility for his life. I am very proud of him!

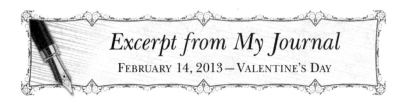

Excerpt from My Journal
FEBRUARY 14, 2013—VALENTINE'S DAY

MY HUSBAND SURPRISED ME WITH A SPECIAL DELIVERY OF OVER twenty pastel-colored roses. They are so beautiful and have filled the house with their fragrance and beauty. I know this was his way of saying, "Thank you for being there for me." This is the man I love!

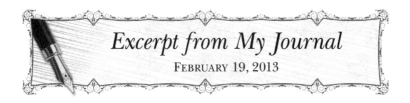

Excerpt from My Journal
FEBRUARY 19, 2013

DEAREST LORD,

Did I thank You for my husband's fifth PSA results with "undetectable level of cancer"? I know we thanked You verbally, but I want to do it now in writing.

Thank You with all our hearts! We thank You for Your blessings on our behalf.

In the months ahead our prayer is that when the testosterone returns to its normal level, my husband's PSA will remain at "undetectable for cancer."

To aid his immune system functioning, he continues his three days of exercise and weight work per week, and we have started juicing organic fruits, vegetables, turmeric, and ginger. I was introduced to juicing by my son, who showed me a video entitled Fat, Sick, & Nearly Dead *by Australian businessman and filmmaker Joe Cross.*

The video is so well done and the information is presented in such an easy-to-understand format that I was inspired to try juicing. My son demonstrated how to do it with his juicer, then I bought one of my own and made my first attempt. I felt like a farmer with all this fresh organic produce on my kitchen counter. The colors of the produce were so vibrant: red, orange, green, purple, yellow.

*It takes a bit of time to wash, core, and cut the produce into pieces that will fit into the juicer, but once that process is completed the juicing is very quick. Most produce does not have to be peeled. The end result is **fabulous!** The juice is multicolored and tastes like fresh spring water. It is absolutely delicious and becomes addictive.*

I showed my husband how to do it, and then he started making his own juice. We both make enough to last one week. Surplus containers can be stored in the freezer. My juice is a 70-to-30 percent blend of vegetables and fruit; my husband prefers a sweeter juice, so his is a fifty-fifty blend. We share samples with each other, like sharing vintage wine.

We choose fruits and vegetables with specific anti-cancer properties and ones that boost the immune system. It is an excellent way to infuse micronutrients into the body—direct and pure— to enhance immune functioning, promote healing, and impede the growth of any rogue cancer cells. It also allows us to consume more fruits and vegetables than we could by eating them.

We started juicing at the same time my husband stopped the Lupron. We are both drinking eight ounces of this special juice per day. We have FAITH that juicing will help him in his fight with cancer. It also aids digestion and gives us radiant hair and skin.

Here is one of our favorite juice recipes:

We use organic fruits and vegetables or produce from our own garden. Rinse each item thoroughly, core fruit of seeds and stems, and sometimes remove the peel as indicated:

2 to 3 pounds of carrots, with or without green tops. No need to peel.

1 bunch of celery, bottom removed, with leafy tops.

3 whole cucumbers, ends sliced off.

2 to 3 whole zucchini, ends sliced off.

2 to 3 small beets, skin peeled, tops and base sliced off.

2 bunches of red Swiss chard, bottom stalks removed. Roll into cigar-shaped bunches and feed into juicer.

2 bunches of purple kale, bottom stalks removed. Roll into cigars.

3 to 4 leafs of collard greens, thick veins removed. Roll into cigars.

Baby spinach, as much as you like.

Several leafs of fresh basil.

4 apples, cored but skin left on. I like to mix Fuji and tart green apples.

3 to 4 pears, cored but skin left on. These add a lot of fiber.

2 inches of fresh turmeric root and ginger, skin peeled or left on.

Sometimes I add half a lemon, but watch the amount as it can be tart.

You may add additional berries and fruits to your liking: watermelon, cantaloupe, oranges, red and dark berries and grapes of any color, pitted peaches and nectarines, etc. I would juice these at a lower speed. I don't use bananas or avocado as they tend to clog the juicer. They can be added later if you blend them in a food processer or blend them with some ice or sorbet or soy milk to make a delicious smoothie.

This recipe provides enough juice for one week, for one person. In terms of juicers, I have found that the inexpensive Breville juicer works very well. It has only seven separate pieces that are easy to assemble and clean.

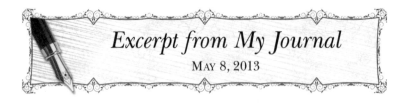

Excerpt from My Journal
MAY 8, 2013

SIXTH POST-RADIATION **PSA: "LESS THAN 0.04 - UNDE-tectable level of cancer"**! *This time **my husband's testosterone had gone up to 359.5**. The normal range is 241 to 827.*

When the medical oncologist gave us the test result he said, **"Delightful!"** *As he was ordinarily pretty reserved, this was quite an expression of happiness and optimism from him. He* *went on to say: "We need to be cautious about the PSA. We will continue to monitor it every three months for a year."*

Both my husband and I have loved working with this doctor. He always sits down with us and takes the time to answer each of our questions. He never gives the impression that he is in a rush. He makes eye contact, smiles, and talks in a gentle, respectful manner. He gives us only as much detail as we are ready to handle. He focuses on the moment and always has a plan of action should the cancer return. He gives us HOPE! We feel safe in his hands.

Dearest Lord, the continued good test results that we received today are wonderful! **I truly believe in my heart that all of the actions we have taken to care for our bodies, minds, emotions, and spirits have enhanced the chances of us getting these results.** *And many people have helped us. Here is a summary of the people and our actions:*

+ *Our urologist who recommended the radical prostatectomy and referred us to City of Hope.*

+ *City of Hope: for the robotic-assisted radical prostatectomy, the combination of dual blockage ADT and radiation—with extra radiation to the enlarged lymph node and continuing Lupron for one year.*

+ *Dietary changes that we made: no beef or lamb, occasional pork, mainly fish, chicken, and turkey. Increase in anticancer fruits and vegetables. Decrease in white flour and sugar, elimination of white potatoes and white rice. No* caffeine (coffee or chocolate) or artificial sweeteners. Little to no alcohol. Stevia as a sweetener. Juicing for the last three months, drinking sixteen ounces of juice per day. Recent gluten-free diet for my husband.

+ The power of prayer and God's intervention on our behalf.

+ Hard workouts combining cardio and weight work, three times a week.

+ The power of love between us.

+ Dealing openly with our emotions and conflict.

+ My husband finding ways to enhance his spirit—through guitar lessons and daily practice, reading books about adventurous warriors, spending special time with his daughters.

+ Both of us acquiring the spirit and characteristics of the warrior.

+ Frequent communication from my son throughout the first year of treatment, whether through phone calls, e-mails, or walks together.

+ The support my husband received from his brother.

+ Fun activities and traditions: family time, movies, concerts and dinner dates, reading time, interesting discussions about current events and our relationship, wonderfully relaxed meals, bonding with Brutie, vacations and new adventures.

+ Both of us working hard in our businesses and reaping the rewards in the form of increased revenues, mental stimulation, and personal satisfaction.

Lord, it seems to be a miracle that we have gotten such good results so far. In going through our paperwork from City of Hope, I found this report written by our medical oncologist on 2-6-12:

> **"He has a lot of unfavorable prognostic factors**, *indicating possibility of at least microscopic metastasis. And looking at salvage radiation therapy nomograms by Memorial Sloan-Kettering Cancer Center,* **the possibility of long-term remission with radiation therapy alone is very low and estimated at 7%. However, with addition of concurrent androgen deprivation therapy the chance of long-term remission increases to almost 30%."**

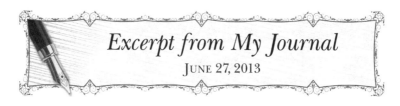

Excerpt from My Journal
JUNE 27, 2013

RESUMED WRITING THE BOOK—CHAPTER 6—AFTER A SIX-month break.

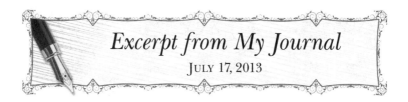

Excerpt from My Journal
JULY 17, 2013

STARTED WRITING CHAPTER 7. MY HUSBAND ASKED ME, "WHY do you have to write this book?" I told him:

"I am writing this book because the whole experience was so hard for us. We didn't know anything about prostate cancer, the treatments, the emotional toll it would take on both of us. It has been an awful experience, filled with so much fear, pain, anxiety, and so many unknowns. There were very few books available to guide us along the way.

If this book can help other newly diagnosed prostate cancer patients and their spouses and significant others, I feel it is my obligation as a wife, educator, and psychotherapist to write it. It is important to make meaning out of our life experiences and offer it to others."

My husband replied: *"I must say, I wouldn't have wanted to go through this without your help. It is still too early to know what is going to happen with me. I am nervous for the next PSA test. We never know."*

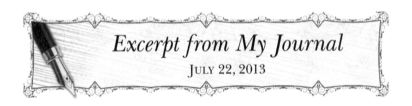

Excerpt from My Journal
July 22, 2013

*Happy to report that **my yearly Pap test came back "normal"**! Thank you, God! My dog Brutie and I leave for New Mexico tomorrow morning for our yearly five-week vacation. My husband will join us for two and a half weeks.*

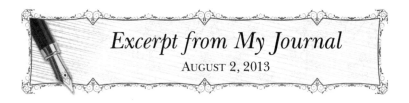

Excerpt from My Journal
AUGUST 2, 2013

MY HUSBAND JUST PHONED ME WITH SOME WONDERFUL NEWS:

"I went for my visit with the radiation oncologist today. He told me I was looking very good, and my blood work revealed that my white blood cell count was at a very healthy level. He did not yet have the results from the PSA test taken earlier this morning.

"He was very pleased to hear that my continence has been restored. I asked him if he thought my erectile functioning would also return. He said, 'You have had surgery, radiation, and hormone deprivation therapy—all of which affect erectile functioning. It may never return. But let's try Viagra and see what happens. Who knows?'

*"I was in my car, driving home, when I got a phone call from the radiation oncologist. He said, '**Your PSA test was undetectable – less than 0.04!** We don't yet know the testosterone level. You will find that out when you see the medical oncologist next week.'*

"He cared enough about me to search out the PSA test results and phone me! Isn't that incredible? I can't think of another doctor who would go to so much effort."

Dearest Lord, once again we are filled with joy and thanksgiving. **This is the seventh post-radiation PSA test that is undetectable for cancer!**

We rejoiced over the phone and reviewed all the actions we have taken in the last year that have supported these results. We are even daring to hope that my husband may be among the 30 percent of those patients with stage T3b who rid their bodies of cancer.

We can only hope and pray and keep on doing what we are doing. The rest is in Your hands, dear Lord. I bid You goodnight.

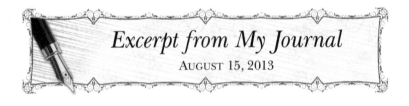

Excerpt from My Journal
August 15, 2013

My darling husband arrived in Santa Fe, and we will spend another two and a half weeks here. Our home provides a spiritual retreat; a place for relaxation, quiet, beauty, healing. We have nothing but free time to enjoy the mountains, the ever-changing sky, walks in the arroyos, the high-desert western landscape and unique adobe architecture, the cultural opportunities, the restaurants, the slow pace of life, each other.

Our days might be lazy (when we eat, sleep, read, and enjoy the monsoon rains in our minka) or hectic (when we attend the exciting festivities of Indian Market).

We will be celebrating our twentieth anniversary on 9-3-13 and are grateful for the gift of all these years together. Thank You, dearest Lord!

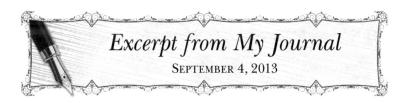

Excerpt from My Journal
SEPTEMBER 4, 2013

I DO NOT FEEL GROUNDED OR MOTIVATED TO WORK OR WRITE *since we are back from Santa Fe. Our twelve-and-a-half-year-old Australian Shepherd, Brutie, was diagnosed with a lumbrosacral lesion that has been growing around his spine and vertebrae for many years. It is now affecting his back legs and hip function, causing pain and restricted movement.*

I am frightened of him becoming old, and of losing him someday. I love him with all my heart and could not bear to see him in a compromised state.

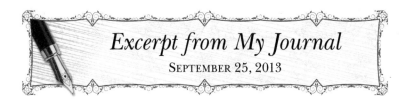

Excerpt from My Journal
SEPTEMBER 25, 2013

DERAILED: THAT IS HOW I AM FEELING. THE NEWS OF BRUTIE'S *lesion on his spine and the chronic pain he experiences have turned my world upside down.*

I try to celebrate the present and find creative solutions to our challenges, but this is cerebral. Inwardly I am reeling on an emotional level. I don't want Brutie to die. I don't want to lose my best friend.

Lord, please help me regain my footing. I think I am making progress, then I fall over or flail. I am often tired, irritable, indecisive. I feel like I am lost.

Please help me find my way back to You—and to my Self. Where is my Self?

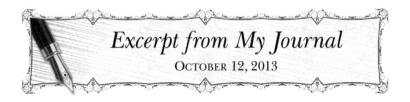

Excerpt from My Journal
OCTOBER 12, 2013

A VERY STRANGE THING HAPPENED TODAY. MY HUSBAND, WHO is normally very calm and gentle, got into this strange mood. He was very irritable and seemed to want to pick a fight with me. He was obsessed about some minor thing I had not done and would not let it go. He kept badgering me. I found myself trying to defend myself, which only made him madder. His voice escalated, his body language was disturbing, and all I wanted to do was get away from him.

The episode was very disturbing to me and caused me to withdraw from him for days. Could this have been caused by his reaction to Brutie's disability, or fears he may have about his cancer and impending PSA test?

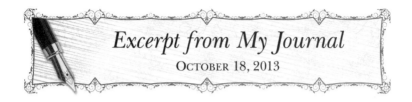

Excerpt from My Journal
OCTOBER 18, 2013

A STORY OF HOPE AND DIVINE INTERVENTION

Tonight, at 8:15 p.m., my husband and I were driving home from dinner. We stopped at a red light. Because it was a warm night my passenger window was rolled down. It was then that I heard the desperate screaming of a cat that was trapped in the sewer, right next to the car.

I told my husband to make a right turn and stop the car so I could take a closer look. I couldn't see the cat, but I began talking to it in a calm voice: "It's okay, we are going to get you out of there. We will be right back."

We drove to the animal shelter, which was closed, then to the closest fire department. I described the emergency to the three firemen, who said they would meet us at that intersection and attempt a rescue. They warned us, however, that it is very hard to rescue cats as they usually run away. I told them, "There is a manhole cover right next to the sewer. I will meet you there. The cat already knows the sound of my voice, and I am good with animals."

We drove back to the cat, and within five minutes a giant fire truck and three kind firemen arrived and were able to pull the cat to safety. They lured it with a chunk of chicken from their dinner. I put the cat in my husband's gym bag and we headed home.

Brutie has always loved cats and wanted one of his own. He was delighted when we brought the cat into the house. He and the cat kissed as if they had always been together. The cat was starving and ate an entire cooked, cubed turkey breast. He immediately settled into a roasting pan that I had covered with a blanket and fell asleep. His body is very thin, and he appears to be one year old. He is a short-haired tiger, with beautiful markings and a sweet disposition.

This rescue seemed to be Divine Intervention. We were in the right place at the right time to rescue this young cat, whom we have named Hope—because it was crying its heart out and pleading to be rescued. I sense we will all be blessed by this event.

Tomorrow I will post a photo and message at the animal shelter to see if there is a worried owner looking for Hope. Who knows how long he was trapped in the sewer and what dreadful experiences he encountered there.

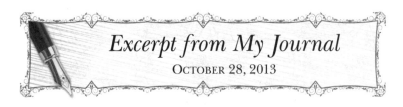

Excerpt from My Journal
OCTOBER 28, 2013

THERE HAVE BEEN NO CALLS FROM THE ANIMAL SHELTER FOR *Hope, and there are no microchips to identify any owner. The veterinarian determined that Hope is a neutered male. We have decided to make him a permanent member of our family as we have all fallen in love with him. He sleeps in the crook of my arm, with his head on my shoulder, kisses my cheeks with his sandpaper tongue, and sometimes shudders with what I call "kittymares"— perhaps nightmares about his life on the streets and in the sewers. He brings joy to me and my husband, friendship to Brutie, and laughter and sweetness to our home.*

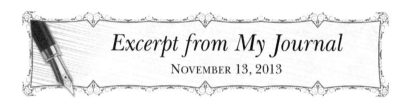

Excerpt from My Journal
November 13, 2013

*Praise God! We met with our medical oncologist and his nurse practitioner today, and my husband received his **eighth consecutive post-radiation PSA test result of "0.04 - undetectable level of cancer."** His testosterone level is 400.3.*

His second bone density test revealed an increase in the bone density in his lumbar spine but a decrease in the bone density in his right hip, with a diagnosis of osteoporosis. The doctor wants him to continue to take calcium supplements and drink orange juice fortified with calcium, along with milk.

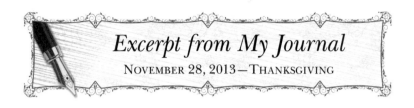

Excerpt from My Journal
NOVEMBER 28, 2013—THANKSGIVING

JUST BEFORE MY HUSBAND AND I WERE TO LEAVE FOR OUR SPE-cial Thanksgiving meal at a hotel in Santa Monica, he came out of the bathroom with a worried look on his face. He said: "I feel a little lightheaded. When I urinated there was a stream of blood mixed with my urine. It filled the toilet bowl." He went on to say: "I have had pink-colored urine for the last couple of weeks, but no burning sensation."

I was very alarmed when I heard this and said, "We need to call City of Hope and see if we can talk to your doctor." My husband allowed me to make the call. I left a message for his medical oncologist, then spoke with a triage nurse. She told me: "Watch to see if there are more episodes. It could be a bladder infection, so have him drink a lot of fluids. If the blood is bright red and there is pain, call us back and we will schedule an evaluation."

My husband hadn't wanted to worry me right before our holiday dinner, so he didn't actually give me these full details until we returned home. I must say that we had a very tense, strained Thanksgiving dinner.

It was my idea not to cook this year, so that I could relax. I had been looking forward to the meal with great excitement and had dressed up for the occasion. We tried to smile and celebrate during the meal, but a heavy dark cloud hung over us.

When we got home my husband told me: "When I first peed blood, it was dark red and I saw a three-inch-long blood clot in the toilet bowl. I didn't tell you about it because I knew you would freak out and it would spoil our dinner. At the restaurant I peed again and it was bright red. When I last peed at 10:30 p.m., it was clear."

I told him that if he had given me the full details, I would never have gone to the restaurant. I said I wanted to call City of Hope with this new information and he said no. I was too frightened to sleep, so I called the triage nurse from the bathroom. She told me to monitor for more episodes and push my husband to drink fluids. She said the doctor would call us in the morning.

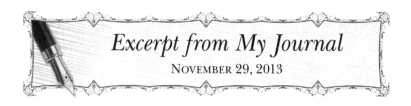

Excerpt from My Journal
November 29, 2013

OUR MEDICAL ONCOLOGIST CALLED MY HUSBAND TODAY. HE said the blood in my husband's urine and the blood clot could have been scar tissue from the bladder, caused by the surgery. The doctor was not too concerned but scheduled an appointment with the City of Hope urologist to evaluate what is going on.

Meanwhile, my husband should pay close attention to any more occurrences.

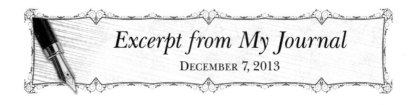

Excerpt from My Journal
DECEMBER 7, 2013

MY HUSBAND HAD ANOTHER UNEXPECTED EPISODE OF EXTREME anger. It came out of nowhere, provoked by an innocent comment I had made. His reaction was way out of proportion to the situation. I was caught totally off guard.

I tried to remain calm, objective, detached. I tried to hold on to my own inner peace. I tried to tell my husband to calm down and asked him what might be causing this anger. Nothing seemed to work. It had to run its full course.

Once again I retreated and tried to comfort myself. I could feel the anger's damaging effect on my body, mind, emotions, and spirit. The only way I could regain my inner equilibrium was to distance myself from my husband for the rest of the weekend. I took long, hot baths; read in my tearoom; took long naps; and spent time outside with my dog.

I had to acknowledge to myself that I was very angry with my husband. More than that, I felt very hurt by his anger. My own anger and hurt lasted several weeks. I found myself not wanting to spend time with my husband. I told him I was very angry, but that did not help the anger go away. The anger and hurt were stuck in my body and psyche.

In an attempt to release them, I scheduled a massage and let out some angry screams in the car just before the massage. No words, just angry sounds. Long, angry sounds. I did not want to scream at my husband. I don't like screaming at people. I prefer to talk about my anger and hurt in a calm voice and express my vulnerable feelings underneath the anger. It feels better on my body and heart. During the massage I did a lot of crying. I told the massage therapist not to worry; that I needed to cry. My body was very sore and tight, and my legs kept cramping with pain that needed to be released. By the end of the massage my body and I were much calmer.

Gradually I regained my "center," and my mind was able to speculate about my husband's anger. Where was this coming from? Why was it happening? Was it because of the blood in his urine? Was he afraid of the cancer returning? Why was he directing it toward me?

This is the theory that I came up with:

Post-Treatment Anxiety Reaction

In the early stages of prostate cancer diagnosis and treatment, fear and anxiety are very strong, normal reactions for the patient and family members. Cancer poses a threat of death and disrupts normal routine. Until all the diagnostic tests and initial treatments are completed, fear and anxiety remain very much on the surface of everyday life.

We feel them, talk about them, and try to cope with these strong emotions.

Once treatment has been completed and patients and their families return to "normal life," the ongoing fear and anxiety about the return of cancer become repressed or pushed down to the level of our unconscious minds. They are out of sight and out of our awareness. **But make no mistake, they are not gone!** Now they live in the dark inner recesses of our bodies, and they have a continued life of their own. Each of these emotions—fear, anxiety, worry, helplessness, dread— generates energy, which cycles through our bodies and attacks vulnerable spots. These emotions cause tension, pain, and unrest in our chests, backs, stomachs, throats, legs, hands. They often disrupt our sleep and digestion and make us prone to illness. They depress our immune systems.

The effect of these repressed emotions is toxic. Sooner or later, like a once-dormant volcano whose molten lava gradually builds up pressure and erupts, the stress and tension build to such high levels that they erupt and spew onto others. The most likely targets are the spouses and significant others of the patient; those who are closest and most trusted. In psychology terms it is called *displaced aggression.*

These eruptions are troubling and baffling to everyone concerned. The patient does not understand why it happens and feels guilty, remorseful, and frightened by these incidents. The family members feel attacked, unsafe, and frightened that it will happen again.

Remembering back to my days as the oncology social worker on the cancer unit, I recall patients having these anger outbursts, which usually spilled onto the nursing staff. Patients sometimes threw their urinals filled with urine, made cutting remarks to the nurses, or complained about the meals or the care they were receiving. The anger was directed toward the nurses because they were safer than the doctors.

The nurses, in turn, would avoid these angry patients at all costs—not answering the call lights, taking their time to bring medications. It became a vicious cycle. As the oncology social worker it was my job to talk with the patient about the anger and try to get to the vulnerable feelings that always lay underneath.

For this reason I caution prostate cancer patients and family members to:

Pay attention to fear and anxiety that are disguised as anger.

It is important to recognize that anger that is out of proportion to the situation is a signal that other, deeper emotions need to be looked at and discussed. The anger is only a symptom that something else is wrong.

A discussion of anger can be a touchy subject. It is an emotion that everyone has, but no one talks much about it. Anger is considered a "bad" emotion, and it makes people uncomfortable. As a society we are not taught how to identify or handle it in a healthy manner. All of us have our characteristic way of dealing with it, which is generally a carryover from our childhoods. Some people do not express it at all but let it eat them up inside. Some people are passive-aggressive. Others are sarcastic. Some people wear a smile to cover their anger while others use food, alcohol, drugs, or other addictive behaviors to avoid it. Some people are quiet, others are loud. Some are aggressive or violent. Others just cry. Very few people can be quietly assertive with their anger.

In most cases, people get angry when they feel they have been violated or when things don't work out the way they had hoped. Anger can be a reaction to helplessness, fear, disappointment, anxiety, rejection.

I have to say that anger is a natural part of the cancer journey. When you think about it, prostate cancer induces many vulnerable feelings: fear of death, fear of the side effects of treatment, fear of loss of sexual ability and continence, fear of loss, fear of the unknown. It causes patients and family members to feel helpless, anxious, and hopeless, adrift in the medical system they do not understand. Cancer is an unknown opponent with deadly powers of destruction.

It is difficult to deal with anger in our relationships because we each have our own way of handling it, which might be quite different than that of the other person. I would say that **anger is only dangerous when it is expressed in a**

manner that frightens, intimidates, or makes the other person feel unsafe.

In my work with clients I use the image of anger being the cork on a bottle, which is filled with vulnerable feelings. To deal effectively with anger, you must take out the cork and see what is inside the bottle. Examining the vulnerable feelings that lay beneath your anger, you can more calmly decide what actions you need to take that will address your needs and those of the people around you.

If you identify that your anger is out of proportion to the situation at hand, I would make the following recommendations:

For the patient:

1. In some type of log or notebook, make a notation each time you have an over-the-top angry outburst. Write the date, the circumstances, and any situations that might have precipitated the outburst. For instance, have you been experiencing any side effects from the treatment? Have you discussed these side effects with your doctor and your spouse/partner? Have you had or are you about to have any tests? Have you been having any disturbing dreams?

2. When you find yourself in the midst of an angry outburst, try to calm yourself down. Even though you are angry, try to lower your voice and refrain from attacking the other person. Move to a quiet space, sit down, and begin doing some deep abdominal breathing.

Relax your face, neck, chest, hands, and abdomen. Breathe in through your nostrils to a count of four, then slowly exhale through an open mouth to a count of four. Feel yourself letting go of anger and tension.

3. As your body begins to relax, ask yourself what might be going on inside you. Are you afraid that the cancer will return? Are you afraid the cancer has spread? Are you afraid your PSA level will climb? Are you afraid your treatment will be unsuccessful? Are you stressed about your work or your relationships? The side effects of the treatment and the changes in your body? Are you overly tired? Have you stopped doing the exercise and activities that would release tension and stress? Are there issues between you and your partner that you have not discussed?

4. When you have calmed down, go back to the person you were angry with and ask for forgiveness for verbally attacking him/her. I know that this may be very hard to do, but it is necessary and will facilitate healing in your relationship. If you do not apologize you will find yourself isolated from the very person who can offer you the most support. Both of you will suffer.

5. Be gentle and forgiving with yourself. Living with cancer is very frightening and anxiety producing. Even after the treatments are completed it is normal to harbor fear and anxiety. They go with the cancer diagnosis. A major characteristic of anxiety is irritability that, left unchecked, can manifest as angry outbursts.

Try to acknowledge these emotions within yourself. Notice them and discuss them with people you trust. After that, concentrate on living your life in the present moment. Savor each day, and continue to take care of your body, mind, emotions, and spirit. Don't worry about what might happen in the future.

6. When you feel anger beginning to build up inside you, try to "nip it in the bud." Notice when you are irritable. Notice the tone and volume of your voice and how you are treating the people you love. Sit quietly with yourself and try to figure out what is going on. Address the underlying issues, the fear, the anxiety straight on. Share your feelings with your loved ones. This is not a sign of weakness; it's a sign of strength.

The way you handle your emotions has a profound impact on your body's ability to fight cancer. Fear and anxiety activate your mid-brain, which releases the stress hormone cortisol along with adrenaline into your bloodstream to enable the fight/flight/immobilization response. The blood vessels in the core of your body become constricted to allow more blood to be directed to your hands and feet so that you can fight or flee from the apparent danger. At these moments, the healing response in your body is turned off. This in turn produces an inflammatory response, which activates cancer cell growth and results in the depression of your immune system.

If you remain in an extreme anger mode, you put your body, mind, emotions and spirit, and your relationships in jeopardy. You are allowing yourself to be controlled by your mid-brain—which is more primitive and reactive than your prefrontal cerebral cortex.

On the other hand, when you take time to reflect on your emotions and calm your body, your prefrontal cerebral cortex (the executive functioning part of the brain) regains control of your body, turns off the fight/flight/immobilization response, releases dopamine (the feel-good hormone) into your bloodstream, and enhances the functioning of your immune system.

For the prostate cancer patient's family members:

I recommend the following coping strategies if and when you are on the receiving end of anger that is out of proportion to the situation:

1. Set boundaries when this anger occurs. Say that it is unacceptable for you to be the target of the anger.

2. Put space between you and the anger. Go to another room. Do not escalate the anger with comments that will fuel the fire.

3. Do activities that will calm you down: naps, hot baths, journaling, praying, meditating, long walks, yoga, exercise, massage/manicure/pedicure, time with a friend or a family member or even a pet to talk about your emotions.

4. Find a way to deal with your own anger and hurt in a manner that is constructive for you. Express these emotions and then try to let them go. I have recently been learning about *tapping*—a method described in the book *The Tapping Solution*, by Nick Ortner. It is a method in which a person "taps" repeatedly on certain acupressure points in the body, with the intention of releasing emotions and stress. I have used this approach on myself and am beginning to use it with clients. I find it to be very effective.

5. Once you have recovered your own "center," take some time to analyze the incident, give plausibility to the "post-treatment anxiety reaction," forgive the patient/your loved one, and slowly come back into contact and discussion with him.

   When you give forgiveness to one another, dopamine is released and "the cycle of love" is re-established.

6. Make a mental note of the frequency of these episodes and pay attention to exacerbating circumstances such as:

   + Fatigue
   + Stress
   + An impending PSA or diagnostic test
   + Side effects of treatment
   + Emotionally disturbing events with family members or pets

Try to give your patient extra TLC (tender loving care) when he is experiencing these issues. It can go a long way in reducing his fear, anxiety, and anger.

7. If the incidents of this level of anger occur frequently, I recommend that both you and the patient go for therapy. Each person in the family must feel safe and respect each other's boundaries. A therapist can help you learn how to do this and can help you investigate what is causing the anger as well as how to deal with all emotions in a healthy manner.

8. Love each other and keep the perspective of the larger picture of your relationship. Cancer is a very frightening illness, which can bring out the worst in each of us. Fear causes us to be angry and irritable. Remember that "perfect love casts out fear." Hold on to each other and cherish your history and memories. Work together to build new memories and happiness. Strive to make each other feel safe and cherished. Don't let cancer destroy your love or your relationship.

Loving one another releases dopamine, a sense of well-being, and enhanced health, according to Bruce Lipton, Ph.D., cell biologist and author of the book *The Honeymoon Effect*.

9. If you yourself experience this same type of anger that is out of proportion to the situation, then follow the recommendations I gave for the patient.

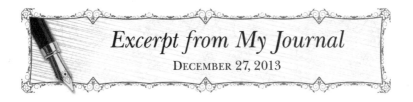

Excerpt from My Journal
DECEMBER 27, 2013

WE WERE SUPPOSED TO LEAVE FOR SANTA FE ON DECEMBER *16, for two weeks, but I made the decision to cancel our trip. I thought it would be too taxing to travel with a new cat and dog, and the stress of the last two months had exhausted me. It had even caused my Lichen Sclerosus to flare up.*

I knew I needed to rest and sensed that a quiet holiday vacation at home would be good for all of us. I must say, it was wonderfully relaxing and fun. We got up late every day, spent the morning in our tea house reading from the book Unbroken *and drinking coffee, then had a beautiful breakfast and leisurely activities. We took naps in the afternoon and often went out for dinner and a movie. My feelings of love and emotional safety with my husband returned, and I really enjoyed his company!*

My handyman and I worked together to install new redwood skylights and roofs to my two tea houses, and we built and installed a miniature redwood Little Free Library in my front yard—to provide a free book exchange for our neighborhood.

The planning, building, staining, and working together outside was medicine for my spirit and body, and I regained my stamina, health, and enthusiasm for life.

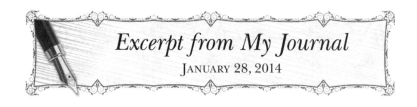

Excerpt from My Journal
JANUARY 28, 2014

As it turns out, God blessed us with rest in December so that we could have the strength to deal with the events that transpired in January:

My husband woke up in the middle of the night in early January with a urinary blockage. *He was very frightened. He was faced with the decision to go to the emergency room at the local hospital or to dilate himself with the catheter his urologist had given him.*

He chose to dilate himself and, as he did it, dark red blood came spurting out every which way, drenching him, the bathroom walls, his pajamas, and the floor in blood. Of course he was very alarmed! We both were. For anyone living with cancer, blood can be a sign that the cancer has spread! The entire toilet bowl was filled with dark red blood and blood clots.

Having cleared the blockage, my husband was now able to urinate comfortably. He left a message for his medical oncologist, put his fears aside for the moment, and was able to enjoy the rest of the weekend.

The following day the doctor called and explained that the blood coming out of my husband's bladder might have been caused by damage to the blood vessels in the bladder at the time of radiation. He went on to say: "Sometimes the bleeding is temporary, sometimes it occurs over a period of time. It will be important to schedule a CT scan of the bladder and then do a scope of the bladder. I do not think the bleeding is caused by any cancer."

On January 8, I took Brutie to see his veterinarian because of his difficulty breathing. For the prior two days his breathing had been labored and loud, making the sound of wheezing or gurgling water.

Brutie was diagnosed with Laryngeal Paralysis *—a neurological disease that affects older, large-breed dogs. Essentially the flaps on either side of the larynx lose their ability to open and close for respiration, eating, and drinking. Brutie required emergency surgery, through a four-and-a-half-inch incision on the left side of his throat, to suture back one of the flaps in an open position.*

Brutie was discharged into my care the following day and has made a remarkable recovery in the last three weeks. Dealing with this life-and-death crisis was enormously frightening and exhausting for me and my husband. Hope hovered close by Brutie's side, sensing something was wrong and giving him support.

Brutie has a good prognosis but will be at risk for aspiration pneumonia for the rest of his life. This requires a total change in his diet. He cannot eat anything that would break into small particles that could then fall into his windpipe and get lodged in his lungs, and he must eat and drink from elevated food bowls.

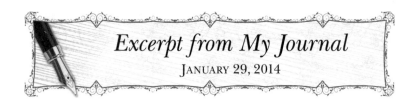

Excerpt from My Journal
JANUARY 29, 2014

MY HUSBAND WENT TO CITY OF HOPE TODAY FOR A CT uro-gram of his abdomen and pelvis. The results showed "no evidence for local recurrent disease." The right obturator lymph node, which had concerned the radiation oncologists at the beginning of radiation, had "decreased in size from 1.6 cm to 0.8 cm."

Thank You, God!

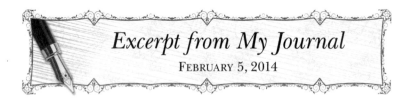

Excerpt from My Journal
FEBRUARY 5, 2014

MY HUSBAND WENT TO CITY OF HOPE TODAY TO HAVE A CYS-toscopy. The procedure was unsuccessful, however, because the urologist encountered a narrowing in the urethra that prevented the scope from moving into the bladder. As my husband was on only local anesthesia and would have been in great pain if the doctor had pushed through the narrowing, it was decided to reschedule the procedure as an outpatient surgery under full anesthesia on February 25.

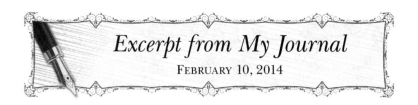

Excerpt from My Journal
FEBRUARY 10, 2014

MY HUSBAND HAD THREE INCIDENTS OF DARK RED BLOOD AND blood clots in his urine today. He called his City of Hope urologist, who asked him to come in for a urine test—to evaluate for infection.

My husband is feeling some anxiety about these recurrent episodes of blood in his urine and is anxious to have the cystoscopy completed.

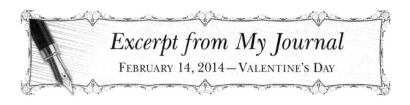

Excerpt from My Journal
FEBRUARY 14, 2014—VALENTINE'S DAY

TODAY WE CELEBRATE ANOTHER YEAR OF HEALTH AND HEALING. Thank You, God, for the gift of another Valentine's Day with my sweetheart!

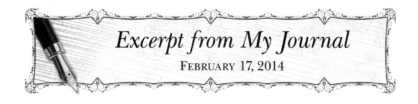

Excerpt from My Journal
FEBRUARY 17, 2014

TODAY WE MET WITH OUR MEDICAL ONCOLOGIST, WHO GAVE *us some wonderful news: My husband's* **ninth consecutive post-radiation PSA test revealed another "less than 0.04 - undetectable for cancer."** *His testosterone is 330.3.*

Here is a summary of the nine post-radiation PSA/testosterone test results:

POST-RADIATION
PSA/TESTOSTERONE TEST RESULTS

TEST DATE	PSA	TESTOSTERONE
4-17-12	<0.04	40.9
5-7-12	<0.04	34.2
7-30-12	<0.04	25.8
11-5-12	<0.04	27.1
2-1-13	<0.04	29.6
5-6-13	<0.04	359.5
8-2-13	<0.04	366.5
11-8-13	<0.04	400.3
2-17-14	<0.04	330.3

We are so very grateful!

Concerning the question of the recurrent blood and blood clots in the urine, our doctor said: "Radiation is the cause of this problem in nine out of ten cases. The radiation burns and thins the blood vessels in the bladder."

It is strangely romantic to be at City of Hope together. We have been coming here for almost two and a half years, and the buildings, hallways, elevators, grounds, the fountain, and the hospital staff are all familiar to us. We have lived through many different emotions and phases of treatment here, traveling from great fear and utter despair to moments of pure elation. We feel safe and very alive here. Our love, though tested, has only increased through this experience.

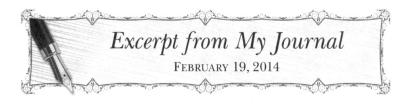

Excerpt from My Journal
FEBRUARY 19, 2014

MY HUSBAND HAD HIS PRE-OP APPOINTMENT TODAY AND WAS cleared for outpatient surgery on February 25.

Our Brutie Boy is doing marvelously well. He is breathing better than he did in Santa Fe this summer, he has increased stamina, and he's enjoying his chunks of raw chicken and raw meat/ground brown rice/baked yam balls. He is energetic and enthusiastic about life again. Praise God!

Brutie receives the same holistic healing approach as all the other family members: prayer, exercise, healthy natural food, massage, soothing warm showers, naps, mental and social stimulation, and tons of love, kisses, and hugs.

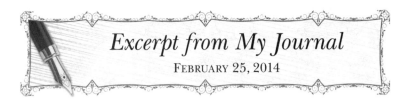

Excerpt from My Journal
FEBRUARY 25, 2014

MY HUSBAND AND I ARRIVED AT CITY OF HOPE FOR HIS OUT-patient cystoscopy this morning. I was allowed to sit with him in the pre-op department. We met briefly with the anesthesiologist, followed by the surgeon.

Both of us gasped when the surgeon said my husband would be going home with a catheter for two and a half days: "I will be removing the obstruction in the urethra, and we use a catheter to prevent the regrowth of the scar tissue." Although the doctor's statement made sense, neither of us liked the idea of the catheter. My husband hated it after his robotic-assisted radical prostatectomy.

The surgeon told us the procedure would take about half an hour and that my husband would be in recovery for two hours afterwards. My husband and I then kissed goodbye, and he was wheeled into surgery.

I decided to wait in my car in the parking lot. This gave me the chance to eat my breakfast in quiet, pray for my husband,

and read. Two hours later I was alarmed when I got a call from the hospital and the nurse told me, "The doctor wants to talk to you." I had expected her to say, "Your husband is out of surgery and you can join him."

I felt the familiar knot of fear hit my stomach, along with a jolt of adrenaline and stress cortisol. I ran into the hospital, up the three flights of stairs, and saw the surgeon waiting for me. "Let's go somewhere private," he said. More fear flooded my body: "Please, Lord, don't let this be bad news."

The surgeon began talking:

"I was able to cut out the obstruction with a little knife. It was devoid of blood, so I cut it until I saw a red margin. When I got into the bladder there were several round red circles: a large one with a blood clot attached, which appeared to be the bleeder, and two smaller ones. I biopsied each of them and cauterized them. We will get the surgical pathology report on Friday, the day your husband comes to have the catheter removed. Expect some bleeding and stinging after the surgery; it's normal.

"In the future it is important to repeat this procedure if your husband has more bleeding from the bladder. Sometimes doctors just assume the bleeding is the result of radiation, and this can have disastrous results if the bleeding is caused by cancer."

Then the surgeon gave me two photos taken inside my husband's bladder, which showed the instrument he used to take the biopsies and the large round red circle. The interior of the bladder looks much like the inside of the colon, and the photos resembled those from a colonoscopy.

My heart and my body relaxed after I talked with the surgeon. I quickly moved to my husband's bedside and was happy to see him looking well but slightly sedated. We waited another half-hour until he was released. Other than a prescription for an antibiotic; some Lidocaine to ease the pain and irritation of the catheter; and the advice to use Extra Strength Tylenol for pain and to call the triage nurse if my husband experienced any fever, excessive bleeding, or nausea, we were not given any further information.

We drove home, happy that the procedure was completed and praying that the biopsies would not reveal any cancer.

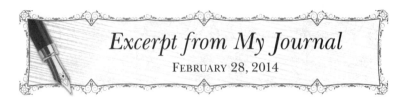

Excerpt from My Journal
FEBRUARY 28, 2014

MY HUSBAND DROVE HIMSELF TO CITY OF HOPE TO HAVE THE *catheter removed and to get the surgical pathology report from the nurse practitioner. He did not meet with the surgeon.*

When the catheter was removed the tip of my husband's penis was very painful. He assumed the pain would go away in a few days.

*The surgical pathology report was negative for cancer: "**no evidence of malignancy**" from the three biopsies. Praise God!*

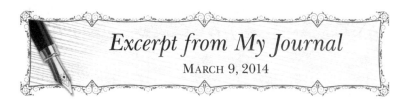

Excerpt from My Journal
MARCH 9, 2014

SINCE THE CATHETER HAS BEEN REMOVED MY HUSBAND HAS experienced some blood in his urine and some stinging when he urinates. These symptoms were supposed to last only a few days, but the stinging continues.

My husband is also experiencing a great deal of pain throughout the urethra, and he has become incontinent. He was not warned that this might happen.

"No one prepared me for the pain or the incontinence. If I hadn't brought a pad when the catheter was removed I would have been totally soaked. I have had to use six to seven pads a day for the last week, and I have so much pain that I am unable to work out at the gym. The urologist told me I should not lift weights until my body has healed. This is all very discouraging!"

My heart breaks for my husband. I feel very sad for him, and helpless. I know his continence is extremely important to him. I remember how hard he worked to regain bladder control after his surgery and radiation. He practiced Kegel exercises every day for months and had to deal with the humiliation of *wearing pads. He was so relieved when it was no longer a problem. Now he has to do Kegel exercises all over again!*

I thought we were in the clear: no cancer in his body and very few side effects from the three courses of treatment. And now this! Incontinence from his cystoscopy? It just doesn't seem fair!

By the same token, however, I acknowledge how very fortunate we are to have no cancer in his body and relatively few serious side effects from the various treatments.

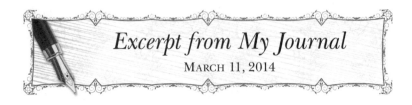

Excerpt from My Journal
MARCH 11, 2014

TODAY MY HUSBAND CALLED HIS SURGEON AND TOLD HIM *about the burning sensation when urinating, the internal pain and soreness in the bowel area above the scrotum, and his incontinence. The surgeon was surprised about the incontinence and could offer no logical explanation for it. In terms of the pain he said, "It should go away."*

My husband felt frustrated after the phone call but vowed to "hang in there" for a while and see if things improve.

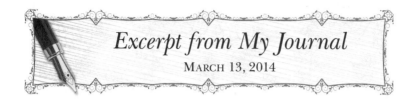

Excerpt from My Journal
MARCH 13, 2014

MY HUSBAND HAS EXPERIENCED DIMINISHED BURNING WHEN *urinating. The flow of his urine, however, has become erratic: "Instead of a normal flow I experience a spray pattern of urination, as if the urethra is partially blocked. Is there an obstruction again?"*

He will wait another week and, if nothing changes, he will call his medical oncologist and discuss these symptoms.

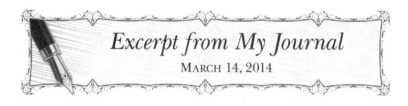

Excerpt from My Journal
MARCH 14, 2014

TODAY MY HUSBAND TOOK BACK CONTROL OF HIS LIFE. *Although he is still incontinent and feeling internal pain in the area of his scrotum, he decided he must return to the gym. He took extra pads and extra underwear and resumed walking on the treadmill and the elliptical.*

"It was important for me to do it. I wanted my life and my body to get back to normal. I wanted to release tension and to experience endorphins once again. I took Advil, which reduced

some of my internal pain. When I got home I was thoroughly soaked, but I did not mind."

I am so very proud of him! He has regained his warrior spirit.

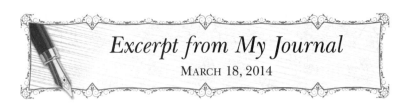

Excerpt from My Journal
MARCH 18, 2014

BUOYED BY HIS SUCCESS AT THE GYM, MY HUSBAND AGREED TO meet a client at a location that was two hours from his office. That would mean a long round trip in traffic and a very long day. Up to now he would have avoided such a trip because of his incontinence.

He planned for the worst and hoped for the best. He took extra pads and underwear. As it turned out, his pad and underwear stayed dry all day until he arrived home.

"I was proud of myself. I am getting my life back. To help with the incontinence I went to the bathroom frequently." I told my husband how proud I am of him and gave him this thought: "Remember, where your mind goes, your body will follow. If you take back control of your mind, your life, your body will try to accommodate you. Positive thoughts and actions generate healing."

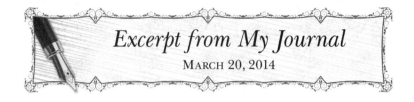

Excerpt from My Journal
MARCH 20, 2014

TODAY I AM SIGNING CONTRACTS WITH MY BOOK PRODUCTION team to begin the editing process for this manuscript and to design the book cover. We are planning for the book to go to press on June 5, 2014. This is a very important day for me.

Obviously I will soon have to stop making entries and come to an ending for this book, which has spanned a two-and-a-half-year period. I wish I could write that we are done with cancer; that my husband is cured and that cancer is a thing of the past. But as I said at the beginning of this chapter, we do not know what is going to happen in the future. That is the nature of cancer and the potential side effects from the treatment. Will we encounter new challenges in our journey with cancer? God only knows. As for us, we must live in present time and savor each new day. We will trust in God; love each other; walk as Four Legs, One Body with the spirit of a warrior; and hold on to hope and determination in our battle against cancer.

Next week my husband and I are invited to be guest speakers for the Advanced Prostate Cancer Group at City of Hope. The group will be expanded to include City of Hope doctors and nurses who treat prostate cancer. This invitation came about because I had given a copy of my manuscript to our medical oncologist and asked him if he would review it. He said he would be delighted to do so.

I was overjoyed when I received his enthusiastic review, which I share with you now:

> *"The thrust of the book is the personal experiences, reflections of a wife of a patient diagnosed with high-risk prostate cancer.*

> *"What is unique about this book are the very specific recommendations on coping with cancer diagnosis, directed to patients, spouses, and healthcare providers. They involve diet, attitude, exercise, hints on how to deal with the 'healthcare system.' It is written from a perspective of a spouse who is also a holistic psychotherapist.*

> *"I would recommend this book to doctors and nurses involved in the care of cancer patients, spouses and significant others of cancer patients, cancer patients, other healthcare providers and social workers involved with cancer care, and other family members.*

> *"The overall message of the book is one of hope and optimism for the cancer patient and the family. It is very honest, talks about the ups and downs, setbacks, fears, frustrations, but ultimately, coping, faith and hope."*

This invitation to speak was a dream come true for me and an answer to my prayer that the sharing of our story might bless other people. The nurse practitioner who runs the group has asked me to address the feelings and concerns of the wives and family members. She wants them to have the opportunity to ask questions and to express what the journey with cancer has been like for them. She also thinks it is important for the patients to hear and understand what their family members have been experiencing.

I am very eager to meet the group members and have the opportunity to share our mutual experiences. With their permission, I plan to include some of their feelings and concerns in the last pages of this chapter. By doing so, this book will truly become *"**Our** **Journey with Prostate Cancer**." I am also eager to hear my husband share his story and hear the questions the patients might ask him. Who knows what will happen? "God works in mysterious ways, His wonders to perform."*

Join me next week. I can't wait!

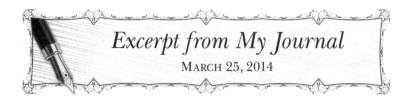

Excerpt from My Journal
MARCH 25, 2014

THERE IS SO MUCH EXCITING INFORMATION TO SHARE ABOUT *our meeting with the Advanced Prostate Cancer Group at City of Hope. It was all that I hoped for and more than I could have imagined.*

The Group Leader

To begin my sharing I will say that the patients and families are very fortunate to have this group—which was the brain-child of the nurse practitioner in the medical oncology department. Through her vision, planning, and dedication she formed the group and worked with her pharmaceutical rep to provide the full dinner at the beginning of each meeting.

This is a woman who goes the extra mile for her patients. She knows it is important to minister to the emotional and psychological needs of the patients and families. She found a way to make it happen. It is very obvious that the patients and wives love her and appreciate her deeply. She is one of them. She sits down beside them and listens to their emotional needs. She plans programs to help them and has found a safe, private space where they can meet. They share an intimate relationship, which is so essential for healing.

Recently, the hospital administration endorsed this pilot group and will provide publicity, social service personnel, and other assistance. It is wonderful when one person can inspire a new program within an organization, and great when adminis-tration will back that program.

The Men

At the beginning of the group I asked, "What do you have to do to qualify for this group?" The men laughed and said that most people would not like to qualify: "You have to have Stage

IV prostate cancer to get in. That means the cancer has spread to other parts of the body."

I knew this group was at a different stage with prostate cancer than my husband. Their prostate cancer is advanced. The whole idea of that scares me. It was so scary that I could not even read about it in the Johns Hopkins White Papers. I didn't want to know about it. Now, here I was with men who had metastatic cancer.

I thank God for this gentle introduction to the concept. These men and women, whom I had come to teach, would be my teachers. We would learn from each other.

*I asked the men how long they have had prostate cancer and there was a wide range of answers: "Since 2005 … 2006 … 2008 … 2011." My heart lifted when I heard this. **These men are the warriors** I had written about in Chapter 6. They have been living with cancer over the long haul.*

I was eager to ask them questions: "To what parts of your body has the cancer spread? What are the various treatments you have been through, and what is your current treatment? What are the side effects of treatment? How scary is it to live with metastatic cancer? How do you handle it? How has this impacted your life and your relationship?"

These brave men gave me hope. They were the embodiment of what our medical oncologist had said to my husband: "If the radiation and the androgen deprivation therapy are not successful in killing the cancer, we have many choices in medications that will allow us to successfully manage the cancer. We have to do this in 70 percent of the cases of aggressive prostate cancer like yours."

To my eyes these men looked great. They weren't in wheelchairs, they weren't on oxygen; they looked like regular, healthy men. And they laughed and joked and were very welcoming to us.

The Wives

The wives were a welcome sight to me. I was so glad they were there, and I was eager to talk to them. We have walked a similar path, one that no one else can fully understand. These women have lived through the diagnosis, the series of treatments, the complications and side effects of the treatments; they have my utmost admiration and esteem. They, too, have been in the battle with cancer over the long haul. I connect and resonate with them, without having to say a word.

As women we are trained from childhood to take care of the members of our families. We are the hub, the heart and soul of the family. I know that these women have instinctively shouldered the emotional burden of their husbands' cancer. The men focus on their cancer, their bodies, their treatments, their jobs, and often do not discuss the emotional aspects of living with cancer. The women pick up the slack for their husbands, worrying, grieving, fearing for them while also handling the day-to-day complications of catheters, the physical side effects of treatment, the doctors' appointments, and the unspoken emotions of their husbands. Meanwhile, they are also running the households, preparing food, taking care of other family members. Most often they do not make time to care for themselves. "Caring for yourself" is not taught to little girls. We are raised to be caretakers of others.

Again, there are so many questions I want to ask the women: "How scary was it when your husband's cancer spread? Are you worrying about the day when the medications might no longer be effective? How has the cancer affected your life as a couple? What do you do to take care of yourself? Have you developed any medical problems as a result of the stress? How has the cancer affected your family? How do you cope with your emotions?"

The Medical Oncologist

Another key member of the group is our mutual medical oncologist. I have mentioned him earlier in this chapter. I don't know of any other doctor who would attend a patient and family group at the end of his busy day, on a regular basis. It is obvious that every one of us loves him. He sits down, cracks jokes, and is intimately connected with each group member on a human level. His face is kind and gentle. He is a concerned human being first, a brilliant doctor second. He never gives up on these patients, and he is available to the family members too. The group members are so comfortable with him that they tease him.

Research data show over and over that the doctor's manner and expectation of treatment outcome have a significant impact on prognosis. We are blessed to have such a wonderful man working at our side to battle the cancer. I believe he is an important ingredient in why these men are doing so well with their Stage IV cancer. He gives us hope and love.

Others Who Attended the Group

Three research/resource nurses also attended the group. They sat down, ate, and mingled with the rest of us. They pored over my Bibliography.

My Presentation

What I decided to share with the group were excerpts from my book, mainly the Prologue and the section of Chapter 6 that talks about patients and families needing to develop the characteristics of a warrior.

Before I began reading I made a few comments to connect myself with the group. I described my husband's cancer and his treatments at City of Hope.

As I spoke about my pleasure in being asked to join them, I began crying. My heart was so happy to finally meet some others on the same journey that I could not hold back the tears. I told them that living with cancer had been very difficult for me. They nodded back in agreement. Many of them had tears in their eyes.

It was fun for me to read my book to a live audience; it is every writer's dream. I eagerly looked at their faces as I read, trying to determine their reactions. Sometimes they laughed, sometimes they nodded their heads; at other times they looked pensive—as if they were considering a new concept or thought. I felt relieved and excited.

When I finished reading, the group made spontaneous comments about themselves and their cancer. The passages I'd read had the desired effect: they helped facilitate group discussion. Praise God! Both the men and women shared. They even asked my husband some questions and joked with him about some of the comments about him in the book: "You're pretty stubborn, aren't you?" "You say no a lot." I was a little worried about how my husband would take these comments, but to my relief he laughed with the group members. I said, "You're going to get me into trouble at home!" and joined the laughter.

I handed out copies of the Bibliography and References and passed around several of the survival books that were referenced on the lists. Everyone was interested in them—both the men and the women. I shared with the group that having my husband read me passages from these books has become one of my favorite intimate activities that we share:

> *"I was never read to as a child. It's something that I regret and envy when others talk about their parents reading to them. So for my husband to make me a pot of hot coffee and read out loud from these exciting and inspiring books, while I relax with Hope and Brutie, is the ulti-*

mate in being cared for. It makes me feel loved and special. It is also a great escape from the cancer and the cares of the day. It inspires us both to be strong, no matter what the odds."

Reactions to the Book

I am happy to report that the entire audience enjoyed my reading and asked when the book would be ready for release. They wanted to buy the book and thanked me for writing it. Some joked, "Will you give us a discount if we buy it from you?" I said, "Of course!" They also asked if my husband and I would return: "We want you to come back and help us."

All in all it was a wonderful experience, and I definitely plan to return to the group as a member and volunteer speaker. Likewise, my husband enjoyed the group and said he would like to return: "When the men were talking I had a lot of questions I wanted to ask them." I thought this was very good. I think my husband can inspire the men and vice versa. They are on the same journey, one that men without prostate cancer cannot understand.

Several of the wives expressed interest in a group for women, one that would be separate from their husbands. I think that would be a good idea. I know that wives and other family members need a forum to discuss their emotions and travails, in a safe place where their husbands would not be worried about them or disturbed by what they express. But I would also like to address some of these issues in the joint group, to facilitate discussion at home.

To this end, I want to close with letters I've written to the patients and their wives/partners.

Letter to the Patients

Dear Gentlemen,

This is a letter written on behalf of your wives/partners. I know you have been very busy with the challenges of living with cancer. I know it has taken all of your strength and attention. And I want to commend you on your achievement.

What I want you to consider today is the role your wife/partner has played in achieving your success. I know that your struggle has been made easier because of her/him. Are you aware of what this journey has been like for her/him? Do you talk about her/his feelings? Do you take time to listen? Are there ways you express your appreciation and love?

As a wife I can tell you that women (and men who are partners) need communication about emotional issues. We have emotional reactions to the cancer and the changes cancer has caused in our family and our life as a couple. We have experienced losses similar to yours. In some ways we, too, are the patients living with cancer. Changes in your bodies have resulted in changes in our intimate relationship. Sometimes those changes leave us feeling unimportant.

Can you try to help us? Can we find new ways to be intimate? We need you to take care of us. We need to feel sexy and appreciated as feminine women (or sexy men). We need your shoulder to cry on. We need to be held and kissed and hugged and celebrated. We need fun activities that take us away from the cancer. We need to get dressed up and have romantic dates. We need flowers or gifts and cards. We need you to be our friend, our confidant, and the man we married so many years ago.

Give us this type of emotional intimacy and we will walk with you anywhere, no matter how difficult the journey. Remember, love is an action *word: Words are nice, but actions are more believable.*

Blessings and love to you,

Judith

Letter to the Wives/Partners

Dear Sweet Ladies/Partners,

I think it might be fair to say that you have been in a "caretaker" role with your man who has prostate cancer. As such, you have probably taken better care of him than you have of yourself. I know that you have experienced a variety of emotions along the way, as well as losses in the way your relationship used to be. I know that your bodies have carried a lot of stress, and your hearts have been burdened. I know that the cancer has taken time and attention from your normal activities and obligations.

I am wondering how you have coped with these demands. What have you done to find support? How do you release fear, anxiety, pain, and stress from your bodies? Have you shared what's going on with your man? Or do you hide these feelings from him in an effort to protect him? What do you need from him? How could he take care of you emotionally and physically? If you are no longer able to have intercourse, are there other forms of intimacy you can think of that will help you two continue to be an intimate couple?

I encourage you to think about these questions; they are vital to your emotional and physical well-being. Further, I encourage you to talk with your man. Help him to grow. Teach him how to take care of you. Be patient with him as he learns. Caring for you will help him in his fight against cancer and will maintain the quality of your relationship.

With love and support,

Judith

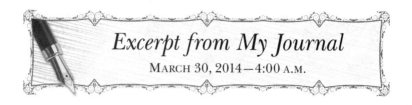

Excerpt from My Journal
MARCH 30, 2014—4:00 A.M.

DEAREST LORD,

I woke up in the middle of the night, agitated. I am concerned for my husband and his current problem with incontinence. It is almost a month since his cystoscopy, and things just aren't right. He still has the internal pain, a split stream or spray when he urinates, scar tissue is building up near the tip of the penis from the catheter, and he is using six to seven pads a day.

We are waiting for the referral to the incontinence specialist but have not gotten a call from the scheduling department. We try to stay peaceful in the present, but it is difficult. Incontinence nags at us. It is an intrusion into our daily lives. It is worrisome to my husband and agitating to me.

I do not feel at peace when there is something wrong with my husband. I am a problem solver by nature, and I cannot fix this problem. It makes me downright angry. How can my husband have lost his continence from a procedure that was supposed to eliminate a urinary blockage? The procedure revealed he does not have bladder cancer, which is a great thing, yet it caused him to become incontinent, which is a bad thing.

You can imagine my husband's dilemma. He doesn't know what this incontinence specialist will recommend. Will he want to do a repeat cystoscopy? Will my husband have to have another post-surgical catheter? Can his incontinence be repaired? All these questions generate fear. We are dealing with the unknown. As his wife who loves him and wants to protect and guard him from harm, my world is off kilter. I don't want my husband to suffer physically or emotionally. It is my nature to analyze the problem and find a solution. I am a problem solver who likes to move quickly: I want to call the doctor, discuss the facts face to face, push for a solution.

My husband moves more slowly. He is willing to be uncomfortable for a longer period, and he will wait for the surgeon's follow-up appointment in three months. He did, however, make two calls requesting to see the incontinence specialist. But if that appointment is not scheduled by next week, I fear he will wait. He often says, "I don't want to be a nuisance or a complainer."

*As I said in the early part of this book, it is my experience that **"the squeaky wheel gets oiled."** When it comes to your life, your cancer, your body—you can't take a back seat. You can't be timid. You should not suffer needlessly. You have to push the medical system to address your concerns! You must be assertive on your own behalf.*

I do understand that there is another possibility going on: that my husband may be reluctant to push for an appointment because he may fear hearing what the problem is. In that case, I have to let him set the pace.

My husband welcomes and relies on my strength. He wants me to come to his medical appointments. He knows I will ask questions and push for solutions. He knows I am assertive on his behalf. Likewise, I know I can count on him to be strong when I am vulnerable. We are a team. We work well together. He is very analytical and has a lot of wisdom. He will do whatever it takes to help me solve a problem or make my heart feel better. He truly loves me and has consistently shown that love over a twenty-year period. It's incredible!

I thank You, Lord, for the gift of my husband. I pray You will bless us once again with Your healing presence. Please help us find a solution to my husband's incontinence and help us deal with the unknown.

LATER THAT DAY:

This has turned into a "state of grace" day—again, one of those days when everything is peaceful and effortless. Having unloaded my agitation in my journal, I was able to express my feelings to my husband rather than be agitated and spoil our day. He, in turn, expressed some of the very same feelings to me. Those feelings had made it difficult for him to sleep as well. We talked openly in a hot bath, starting the day with warmth and relaxation, and encouraged each other. We vowed to press for a solution to this incontinence problem. Our spirits were lifted, and we were a united front.

Then we took Brutie to the park and had a fun walk in the sun. When we got home we had reading time and my hot coffee in the tea house, followed by a really good breakfast.

The rest of the day flowed perfectly: My husband practiced guitar, then gave me a concert. I spent time writing, then shared what I had written. We ended the day by bringing in Indian dinner and watching our favorite Sunday-night television shows. It's amazing how asking God for help can turn things around.

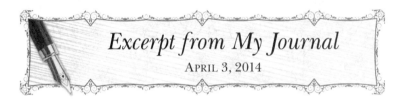

Excerpt from My Journal
APRIL 3, 2014

THIS IS THE LAST ENTRY FOR MY JOURNAL. BECAUSE THE TITLE *of this book is* Our Journey with Prostate Cancer *I would like to conclude with a brief interview with my husband. The basic question I asked him to address:* **"What changes have you made in your life because of the cancer?"**

His response:

> *"I brought more balance into my life. Before cancer I was too one-dimensional, mostly focused on work and family. I didn't make special time for myself. I didn't have any hobbies and had few outside interests, other than attending cultural events, movies, and entertainment.*

Specifically, I have made the following life changes:

1. *Changes to diet. Gave up most sources of caffeine (regular coffee, chocolate, tea, cola drinks, etc.). Stopped drinking sodas with artificial sweeteners (aspartame, Splenda, and sucralose) and switched to sodas sweetened with Stevia, which is a natural plant-based sweetener. Eliminated most red meat and increased the amount of fish, poultry, fruits, and vegetables. Started juicing with organic vegetables and fruits to supplement meals. Eliminated major sources of wheat gluten. Cut back on fried foods and desserts. Added daily probiotic supplement to improve digestion and bolster immune system. The results of all these changes: healthy blood chemistry, weight loss to optimum for body type, elimination of headaches, improved resistance to colds and viruses, and reduced side effects and recovery time from cancer treatments.*

2. *Started weekly lessons to learn classical guitar, a long-term goal of mine. I made a serious commitment to become the best musician I was capable of.*

3. *Started a two-days-per-week exercise regimen of cardio and weight work. That was later expanded to three days per week.*

4. *Started reading real-life adventure books featuring survival against the most challenging of conditions*

(*Into Thin Air, Unbroken, Endurance: Shackleton's Incredible Voyage, etc.*).

5. *Began taking daily "breaks," even naps at times, during the workweek (where possible). These have become special moments, without feelings of guilt.*

6. *Started going to bed earlier, resulting in longer, more satisfying sleep.*

7. *Changed eating habits: eating dinner earlier and eliminating late-evening snacks.*

8. *Began taking early-evening hot baths, which are for relaxation and are also soothing for any cancer-treatment discomfort.*

9. *Started focusing more on the present and trying to enjoy each and every day.*

10. *Became more flexible and open to change, which has eliminated a measure of stress in my life."*

In a similar fashion I will answer this question: **"What have I learned from our journey with prostate cancer?"**

1. **Humility.** *Prior to my husband's prostate cancer I prided myself on being a "strong" person. Throughout my life I have weathered many obstacles and challenges. I have learned to incorporate a variety of self-care skills to help keep my life in balance and health. I was "strong" in body, mind, emotions, and spirit.*

*The journey of living with my husband's prostate cancer, however, has been the most frightening and challenging experience of my life, and it has had a profound impact on my **body**. I was totally unprepared for the fatigue, compromised immune system, and medical problems that I experienced. **Emotionally and psychologically** I was extremely challenged to deal with the fear, loss of control, and anguish that go along with living with cancer.*

2. ***My spirit*** *has been extremely challenged by our journey with prostate cancer—many times feeling overwhelmed by fears of death and loss, and physical fatigue. However, I've learned that my relationship with God is the same as always. Each time I have cried out to Him, my spirit has been strengthened and renewed, and a sense of peace and hope has returned to my body. I have never developed a deep depression or suffered a panic attack.*

Throughout my life I have reached out to God, and He has taken care of me—giving me courage, peace, hope, direction, insight, love, and healing. I do believe that He has assisted and is assisting my husband in his battle with prostate cancer. We have experienced an ease of scheduling treatments, relatively minor side effects of the treatments, and the absence of post-treatment PSA, so far—all of which feel like divine intervention. And we experience peace and hope in the present.

3. *I've learned how very much I love my husband and how precious he is to me. We have been challenged, to be sure, but our love is stronger and sweeter than ever before.*

4. *I've learned that there have been exciting medical advances and research in the treatment of cancer over the last thirty-five years. So much more is known about cancer cells and their vulnerability. A greater number of treatment options exist that allow people to manage their cancer.*

   Likewise, so much more is known about the body's immune system and the role of NK cells, as well as the impact of diet, meditation, prayer, exercise, mental attitude, and emotions. **I am more convinced than ever about the importance of a holistic approach to treating cancer.**

5. *I have learned that the loved ones of the prostate cancer patient suffer as much as the patient. It's as if we both have cancer. The cancer affects both of us, in our bodies, minds, emotions, and spirits. As such, both of us need attention and care, love and support.*

6. *I have learned the importance of family and friends and how much they are needed when we are living*

with cancer. We cannot do it by ourselves. We are vulnerable, tired, frightened, and we need to be lifted up, encouraged, and loved.

Reflections

WE HAVE WALKED THROUGH THE VALLEY OF THE SHADOW of death and come out the other side. My husband was diagnosed with a very aggressive, high-risk form of prostate cancer on November 11, 2011. He was a clinical Stage III (T3-b) and had a very poor prognosis. He had a 70 percent chance of recurrence of the cancer, even with robotic-assisted radical prostatectomy, radiation, and dual blockage androgen deprivation therapy.

I believe that the "Story of Hope and Divine Intervention" involving our cat Hope (see my October 18, 2013 journal entry) serves as a parable about our journey with cancer. We prayed, cried out, and asked God to help us. The Spirit was with us every step of the way, guiding our path, leading us to the best treatment team at City of Hope, giving us discernment about the treatment choices, and inspiring us to take charge of our battle with cancer by implementing specific strategies for our bodies, minds, emotions, and spirits.

Our journey with cancer has been a continuation of our love story. Married for twenty years now, my husband and I have been through many trials, challenges, and losses. I would say that our experience with cancer has been, by far, our biggest and toughest challenge. But you know what? It has also led us to our greatest joy, learning, and bonding as a team. We couldn't have gotten through this without each other. We have made many changes to our lifestyle because of the cancer, and they have benefited both of us and our families. And we have been blessed with the opportunity to help and bless other people living with prostate cancer.

At this point we are both healthy, very happy, and prospering in our careers. This June I will be teaching a workshop entitled "Mindfulness on the Cancer Unit: Acknowledging Our Fears and Allowing God to Work" at the Ninth Annual North American Conference on Spirituality and Social Work in Fredericton, New Brunswick. I am hoping this is just the beginning of my international speaking engagements. I believe that God wastes nothing; that He uses every experience we have for the greater good.

I close with the prayer that you and your family will be blessed, guided, and empowered on your own journey with prostate cancer. It has been an honor to come into your lives. I send you our love and appreciation, and I would be so happy to hear from you. You can be my teachers. Remember: It is *Our* **Journey with Prostate Cancer!**

References and Other Reading Material

(in chronological order as they appear in the book)

References

Introduction

Getting Well Again: A Step-by-Step, Self-Help Guide to Overcoming Cancer for Patients and Their Families, by O. Carl Simonton, M.D., Stephanie Matthews-Simonton, and James L. Creighton, Bantam Books, 1978.

The Healing Journey: The Simonton Center Program for Achieving Physical, Mental, and Spiritual Health, by O. Carl Simonton, M.D., and Reid Henson with Brenda Hampton, Bantam Books, 1992.

Prologue

Creating A Healthy Life and Marriage: A Holistic Approach: Body, Mind, Emotions and Spirit, by Judith Anne Desjardins, LCSW, BCD, MSWAC, Chapter 5, pages 93-94, Spirit House Publishing, 2010.

Chapter 1

Daily Word, by Silent Unity—(800) 669-7729 or *www.silentunity.org.*

Links for research on the effects of prayer on health:

www.cancer.org/treatment/treatmentsandsideeffects/complementary andalternativemedicine/mindbodyandspirit/spirituality-and-prayer

www.ncbi.nlm.nih.gov/pubmed/22894887
archinte.jamanetwork.com/article.aspx?articleid=485161
onlinelibrary.wiley.com/doi/10.1002/pon.1129/abstract

Chapter 2

Prostate Cancer Research Institute (PCRI),
Helpline: (800) 641-7274; *www.prostate-cancer.org*; info@pcri.org.

Chapter 3

American Joint Committee on Cancer Staging Manual, sixth edition,
American Joint Committee on Cancer, 2002.

The 2005 International Society of Urological Pathology (ISUP)
Consensus Conference on Gleason Grading of Prostatic
Carcinoma, *American Journal of Surgical Pathology*, *29*(9): pp.
1228-1242, by J.L. Epstein, W.C. Allsbrook, Jr., M.B. Amin,
et al, 2005.

Anticancer: A New Way of Life, by David Servan-Schreiber, M.D.,
Ph.D., pp. 36, 40, Viking Penguin, 2009.

*Life Over Cancer: The Block Center Program for Integrative Cancer
Treatment,* by Keith I. Block, M.D., Bantam, 2009.

The Living Bible, Psalm 40: 1-3, Tyndale House Publishers, 1971.

The Willpower Instinct, by Kelly McGonigal, Ph.D., Penguin, 2012.

Chapter 4

www.kegel-exercises.com

Chapter 5

The Living Bible, Psalm 116: 1-13, Tyndale House Publishers, 1971.

Chapter 6

National Comprehensive Cancer Network Clinical Practice Guidelines in Oncology, Prostate Cancer, Version 4.2011.

"Is There a Standard of Care for Pathologic Stage T3 Prostate Cancer?" by Ian M. Thompson, Catherine M. Tangen, and Eric A. Klein, published in the *Journal of Clinical Oncology,* June 20, 2009, Vol. 27, No. 18, (pp. 2898-2899).

"Preventing and Treating the Side Effects of Testosterone Deprivation Therapy in Men with Prostate Cancer: A Guide for Patients and Physicians," by Brad Guess, edited from *PCRI Insights,* November 2007, Vol. 10, No. 4.

"Radiotherapy Combined with Hormonal Therapy in Prostate Cancer: The State of the Art," by Piotr Milecki, Piotr Martenka, Andrzej Antczak, and Zbigniew Kwias, published in *Cancer Management and Research,* October 11, 2010, Vol. 2 (pp. 243-253).

"Prostate Disorders: Your Personal Guide to Prevention, Diagnosis, and Treatment," by H. Ballentine Carter, M.D., *The John Hopkins White Papers,* page 37, 2011.

National Cancer Institute website: *www.cancer.gov/cancertopics/pdq/treatment/prostate/Patient/page2.*

Women's Bodies, Women's Wisdom: Creating Physical and Emotional Health and Healing, by Christiane Northrup, M.D., Bantam Books, 1998.

Endurance: Shackleton's Incredible Voyage, by Alfred Lansing, Basic Books, 2007.

The Endurance: Shackleton's Legendary Antarctic Expedition, by Caroline Alexander, Alfred A. Knopf, 1998.

Frozen in Time: An Epic Story of Survival and a Modern Quest for Lost Heroes of World War II, by Mitchell Zuckoff, HarperCollins Publishers, 2013.

Unbroken: A World War iI Story of Survival, Resilience, and Redemption, by Laura Hillenbrand, Random House, page 148, 2010.

Chapter 7

The Living Bible, Zachariah 4:6, Tyndale House Publishers, 1971.

Wheat Belly: Lose the Wheat, Lose the Weight, and Find Your Path Back to Health, by William Davis, M.D., Rodale Books, 2011.

www.fatsickandnearlydead.com

The Tapping Solution: A Revolutionary System for Stress-Free Living, by Nick Ortner, Hay House, 2013.

The Honeymoon Effect: The Science of Creating Heaven on Earth, by Bruce H. Lipton, Ph.D., Mountain of Love Productions, May 2013.

www.littlefreelibrary.org

Other Reading Material

Super Immunity: The Essential Nutrition Guide for Boosting Your Body's Defenses to Live Longer, Stronger, and Disease Free, by Joel Fuhrman, M.D, HarperCollins, 2011.

Prostate Cancer and the Man You Love: Supporting and Caring for Your Partner, by Anne Katz, Rowman & Littlefield Publishers, 2012.

The Prostate: A Guide for Men and the Women Who Love Them, by Patrick C. Walsh, M.D., Johns Hopkins University Press, 1995.

Dr. Patrick Walsh's Guide to Surviving Prostate Cancer,
by Patrick C. Walsh, M.D., Warner Books, 2001.

How We Survived Prostate Cancer: What We Did and What We Should Have Done, by Victoria Hallerman, Newmarket Press, 2009.

Making Love Again: Hope for Couples Facing Loss of Sexual Intimacy, by Virginia Laken and Keith Laken, North Star Publications, 2002.

The Lovin' Ain't Over: The Couple's Guide to Better Sex After Prostate Disease, by Ralph Alterowitz and Barbara Alterowitz, Health Education Literary Publishers, 1999.

The Healing Journal: Taking Control of Your Journey Through Cancer, by Lynda Peterson, Lynda Peterson, 2011.

Grace Like a River: An Autobiography, by Christopher Parkening with Kathy Tyers, Tyndale House Publishers, 2006.

Links for Erectile Dysfunction

www.medicinenet.com/script/main/mobileart.asp?articlekey=395
Erectile Dysfunction (ED)
What is erectile dysfunction?
What causes erectile dysfunction?
What are the risk factors for erectile dysfunction?
How is erectile dysfunction diagnosed?
What is the treatment for erectile dysfunction?
What is the prognosis for erectile dysfunction?

www.medicinenet.com/script/main/mobileart.asp?articlekey=24721
Erectile Dysfunction (Impotence)
Take the Impotence Quiz
Impotence Slideshow
Sex-Drive Killers

Index

About the Author

WITH LISTINGS IN WHO'S WHO IN THE WORLD, WHO'S Who in America, Who's Who in Medicine and Health-care, and Who's Who in American Women, Judith Anne Desjardins has maintained a thirty-six-year holistic psychotherapy practice. As an educator, she has taught nationally and in Canada, and her first book, *Creating A Healthy Life and Marriage*, is the winner of sixteen book awards in the United States and Canada. A Polish translation was released in 2013.

She is a Licensed Clinical Social Worker, a Board Certified Diplomat in Clinical Social Work, and a Master Social Work Addictions Counselor.

Judith Anne Desjardins is available for consultations, workshops, and speaking engagements.

For information regarding her availability, please visit: *www.judithannedesjardins.com* or *spirithousepub@verizon.net*

To purchase additional copies or for information about special discounts for bulk purchases, please visit *judithannedesjardins.com*.

A portion of the sale from each book will be donated to City of Hope Prostate Cancer Research.